Father Caesar,
May God bless you and your ministry to his people. I cannot thank you enough for what you have done for us!

Whispers & Roses

A Journal of Healing from Cancer

Diana Fidone Griggs

Diana Fidone Griggs

Inner Light Productions

Helotes, Texas

Whispers & Roses

A Journal of Healing from Cancer

Published by Inner Light Productions
11731 Drought Pass, Helotes Texas 78023, USA
Phone: (210) 363-8647 Fax: (210) 695-5756
Email: ilp@satx.rr.com

Printed and bound in the United States of America

Cover Design by Alexandra Cerovac, Zagreb, Croatia
Printed by Litho Press, Inc., 4334 Milling Road, San Antonio, Texas 78219

ISBN 978-0-9842-9490-9

Published in the United States of America

This book is dedicated to my loyal and sweet husband Lloyd, my up-lifting and loving daughters Angela and Andraya, supportive parents Luciano (Louis) and Donna Fidone, and to the thousands of people who suffer needlessly with cancer.

Disclaimer

The author of this book is not a medical doctor and does not claim to have the knowledge and expertise of a medical doctor. No portion of this book may be construed as medical advice, but simply a recounting of the healing process encountered by an individual. Each person has uniquely different needs and it is recommended that if you have symptoms of a medical condition, you seek the advice and care of a physician.

The material presented is for educational and spiritual purposes. The author also does not claim to be a theologian or a theological expert, but only a small vessel of the Lord. You are still encouraged to seek out a flock of fellow believers and a pastor/reverend/priest/rabbi, etc., who can serve as additional beacons of light.

All efforts have been made to present the truth as researched, but the author is not responsible for the guaranteed accuracy of the sources used. This book is by no means exhaustive and totally inclusive of every type of treatment, product, and service available.

Many products mentioned in this book are not approved by the FDA (Food and Drug Administration) as treatments for any sort of disease, except for the chemotherapy drugs mentioned. Any mention of alternative products used is to illustrate those used by the author and are not necessarily recommended for each person. You are encouraged to do your own research. The intent is to indicate that there are other choices in all areas and each person must explore these on their own.

Some names have been changed to respect the families involved and to protect their privacy. Every journal entry is not shown, but only those that related to the topic and healing.

Table of Contents

Introduction

This endeavor started as a journal, written for my family and myself, of recovery from a serious cancer diagnosis. I began to receive messages and encouragement from the Lord, and upon the crazy suggestion from my friend Phil Raymond to write a book, I realized that the messages I heard needed to be shared with the rest of the world. The book is organized around my journal entries, which are assigned no given year because they are timeless. Most chapters contain physical information to understand the workings and non-workings of the body, as well as mental information. And most importantly, spiritual enlightenment and saving grace is included in the **bold** lettering of the Lord's words.

There were days when I wondered how anyone survived the ravages and bludgeoning of chemotherapy. I learned what it felt like to be dying slowly from the inside. But, I was also fortunate enough to feel the life force returning and becoming stronger than it had been in years.

Merely surviving a deadly disease is not enough. I intended to survive and thrive. That is what we are meant to do. The hardest part for me is that when I meet people who are suffering, I know that it doesn't have to be that way for them or their loved ones. Because there was an answer out there for me, I know there is an answer out there for you or someone you know. This book shows you how I discovered the answers and am still discovering information that can assist others in recovering from cancer or any other disease.

Along with physical healing came spiritual healing. This book follows my prayers, innermost thoughts, and intimate conversations with the Supreme Being and the Son of God. The incredible love of the Lord, that I had doubted really existed for me, was revealed in the most heart-touching and beautiful way and yet, it is still difficult to fathom. I do not feel any more special than the next person, but

I am very grateful for all revelations, insights, and demonstrations of love brought to me in an extreme measure through many different avenues.

One of my favorite relaxing things to do is to feed the birds in my back yard and to sit and observe them. They have taught me much. There is one I identified with for awhile that I nicknamed "floppy". A predator had claimed his tail feathers, so every time he walked, he flopped over sideways and would fight like crazy to right himself so he could go after food. That's what I felt chemotherapy did to me...took my tail feathers and left me flopping around, trying to walk. Only God's grace could set me upright again and allow me to fly. God gave me the means to the wholeness of body and spirit and this is my story......

Author's Note- Some Scripture references are taken from the The New American Bible for Catholics which contains extra-canonical books not found in Protestant versions.

Prologue

About six months before this story began, my cat, Snickers, was attacked by another cat in the neighborhood. A few mornings later, I came down the stairs for breakfast and noticed that he wouldn't eat or drink, and could hardly move, much less walk. I quickly rushed him to the local animal hospital and waited anxiously for the doctor to come in. After a thorough examination, she informed me that apparently he had been scratched or bitten by another cat and that he had an infection. She gave him an injection of a few cc's of water under the skin and an antibiotic pill. She gave me several of the antibiotic pills and I was instructed to make sure that he received a pill each day for the next several days.

After I took him home, his condition was better but he was still gravely ill. He would not eat or drink so how could I get that pill down him? The following day, I bought some canned food and put the pill in it. He wouldn't eat it. I finally forced it down his throat with some of the food. A little while later, he threw it back up with the food. He was still lethargic, barely moving, and not eating or drinking well at all. I made several attempts to get that pill down him. He threw everything back up and continued to throw up. I called the animal hospital and explained my plight. "Is there another medicine I can give him?" I asked desperately. "This one is making him throw up!" The attendant checked with the veterinarian who then came on the line. I told her the same thing and she said there was no other choice because that was the medicine usually prescribed and to just keep trying. Was my cat going to die? What could I do? I was very afraid that I was going to lose him.

Later that day, the house was silent and my husband was at work. I literally got down on my knees in my bedroom closet and prayed fervently for Snickers. I cried out to the Lord to help me get that medicine down him and for it to work. A small voice seemed to answer me in my head, almost like a thought. The message was this, "**Have no fear. I will heal him. Do nothing further.**" Was I talking to myself? Did my brain play a trick on me? Who was that putting thoughts in my head? Was this some evil entity trying to trick me into letting Snickers die?

I prayed, "Lord, is this you talking to me? How will I know this is REALLY you? The message came into my head, "**Wait and see if what I have said comes to pass. Have faith.**" I was definitely in frightening territory. I'd never before heard any kind of "voice" and never been asked to have faith. I thought I was going crazy while I looked at my poor sick cat. What if I did nothing and he died? How could I live with that? So, I prayed more and I waited. I didn't give him any more medicine. In fact, I did nothing.

The next day, I anxiously arose in the morning to go and check on the cat to see if he had made it through the night. Not only did he make it through the night, he was perfectly healthy, back to his old self, eating and drinking and ready to play with his cat toys. It was truly a miracle as far as I was concerned. The unused pills lay on the counter. God had actually SPOKEN to me! I had actually LISTENED! At that time, I didn't tell anyone about this entire experience.

My cat is still healthy and doing well. Thanks be to the Lord.

1
Shock and Awe

The Bad News

Sitting in the doctor's waiting room in my "fat" jeans, I anxiously awaited the results of an abdominal CAT scan from a few days ago. The doctor had called and asked me to come in to review the results, which wasn't a good sign. This shouldn't be happening, I told myself. I'm retired from school administration, happily selling real estate, teaching at the local university, and looking forward to more travel.

The nurse called me in to the vital signs area to weigh me. The scale said 140! I usually weigh 125, but in the past couple of years I had gained weight. What started off as a little pouch was now a protruding swollen abdomen. I was wearing size 12 pants (up from size 6) and even those had gotten tighter. The doctor entered with a sympathetic look on his face that told me much more than words.

"Hello, doctor."

"Good morning, Diana. Is your husband with you?"

Why would my husband be with me, I thought? It's not as if I dragged him around to all of my doctor appointments. This was my first confirmation that something was amiss.

With a somber face he stated, "We have the results of your CAT scan and they don't look good."

"What do you mean, they don't look good?" I think at this point, it was still just an annoyance to me. "I know I get migraine headaches, have acid reflux, allergies, and some fatigue, but what could this be? Is it a cyst? Do I have an intestinal problem?"

"I'm afraid not," he said, "You have stage 3C ovarian cancer."

"Cancer? Are you sure? Could there be some mistake?"

"No, it's certain."

I was stunned. A year ago, I went to the gynecologist who told me I'd gained 7 pounds in a year and that I needed to watch what I was eating. This doctor was informing me that it was the dreaded "C" word that strikes fear in everyone who even hears it spoken. "What does stage 3C mean?" I asked.

"It means that the cancer has spread throughout your entire abdomen," he replied sadly.

"Is that why I look pregnant?" I'd already had a partial hysterectomy years ago and was menopausal, so I thought it was just from eating too much and not exercising enough.

"Yes, it's a secondary result of the cancer. The cancer cells create a build- up of fluid called ascites. Your abdomen is full of it and that is contributing to the swelling."

"No wonder my abdomen is so big, and all this time, I thought it was fat settling around my waist and abdomen." Then I asked, "How many stages are there?"

"There are 4 stages and 3 sub-stages. The sub stages are labeled a, b, or c depending on the amount of involvement," was the reply. Stage 1 is localized and stage 4 is spread to other places, including the lymphatic system.

"So, stage 4 the worst?"

"Yes."

"So, stage 3C is pretty bad?"

"I'm afraid so. It means that even though it started in your ovaries, it has now spread to other nearby organs. We won't know how badly unless we get inside and take a look." This was serious and I got a sick feeling in the pit of my stomach. My acid reflux was definitely acting up at this moment.

"What are my options, doctor? Can it be removed or is it inoperable?" I was so afraid that he'd say that it was hopeless—inoperable—go plan the funeral.

"Yes, it is operable and you can have much of it surgically removed which is called de-bulking."

"Then, I want that done as soon as possible."

"I know the name of a good surgeon. Let me see if I can get him on the phone." He left the room and I waited. How could this diagnosis be possible? I thought that I ate fairly well (although I did have a sweet tooth), exercised at the gym (although not as often as I should), and had just started an exciting new phase of my life. Did they get my results mixed up with someone else? This just couldn't be true, I told myself. Now, I understood why hiring a dietician and a gym trainer to work with me had produced no results. A short while later he re-entered the exam room.

"Well, I talked to the surgeon. He's available to do surgery next Friday."

"Whoa! That soon? Alright, let's get on with it. I want this cancer gone from me."

"Ok, I'll call him back and schedule the surgery. Here's his name and number. Call him when you get home and set up an appointment. He also wants you to have a colonoscopy before the surgery."

"What for? I just had one a few months ago and I hate those things!"

"He wants to see if the cancer has spread into your intestines."

"Oh, doctor, I hope not. This bad news is more than I can handle right now. Anyway, I need time to think."

"I know it is a big shock to you and it is to me as well. I wish you well with everything."

I remained in his office for an hour, asking questions, trying to grasp what he had told me, and yet not wanting to accept it.

In a daze driving home from the doctor's office, watching all of those other drivers on the road with me, I wondered, "Did any of you just get devastating news like me? Are you going shopping, going to work, or heading somewhere to visit a friend—anything mundane? Do any of you people know what I've just been told? This is SO unfair!" *My grief is incurable, my heart within me is faint. (Jeremiah 8:18)* I screamed inside the safety of my car where no one could hear. I somehow made it home but I don't remember the drive. The minute I walked into the house, my husband Lloyd read my face as I started to cry and told him the devastating news. We cried and hugged each other in what seemed to be a night marish dream. Seeing my husband cry was probably the hardest part at that moment. In our 12 years of marriage, I only saw him cry one time and that was when he had to put his dog Heidi to sleep. It was comforting to know that I at least ranked as high, or higher, than his beloved pet, but it didn't take away the absolute paralyzing fear and panic overtaking me at that moment. *Like a swallow I utter shrill cries; I moan like a dove. My eyes grow weak, gazing heavenward: O Lord, I am in straits; be my surety! (Isaiah 38: 14)*

Just last week, I took my friend Maggie to the cancer center for a cancer treatment. She originally had breast cancer and had undergone chemotherapy six years ago. Now, another tumor had come back, this time in her lungs. I had walked in with her, wondering how she had the strength to undergo chemotherapy for the second time in her life. The faces I saw in that treatment center as we entered were devoid of hope and no one spoke to anyone else in a big room full of chairs and IV poles.

I had watched horrified, as the treatment nurse tried to find a vein and had a difficult time getting Maggie's IV started. We sat and talked during the treatment for 3 hours, watching them change one empty bag of liquid for another bag of some other fluid. My thought was, "Oh, Lord, I hope I never have to go through that." It also brought back a childhood memory of my friend Kathy from grade school who had a grandmother dying of cancer living with her family. I used to think that people who got cancer were lucky because they knew when their time was coming and they had time to repent of all of their sins. No unexpected dying for me. Now, with this diagnosis, it seemed like such a cruel twist of fate. I can't believe I had thought that way as a child. Had this disease invaded my body to grant me my wish? Had I asked for this? What was I thinking? How had my understanding of God allowed me to wish such a thing upon myself?

My sister Joann had called two months previously to tell me that her husband, Myron, had been diagnosed with esophageal cancer and was getting ready to undergo chemotherapy and radiation. Darkness and disease seemed to be surrounding me everywhere I turned. *My dwelling, like a shepherd's tent, is struck down and borne away from me. (Isaiah 38:12)*

Get It Out of Me

The next week went very quickly, with lab tests and x-rays. How interesting that they had to make sure my body was in good enough shape for surgery. One thing was certain. My immune system had been compromised or these abnormal cells would not have been allowed to grow in the first place. I was beyond scared. I was in the panic mode. This just couldn't be happening to me. I had so much to live for. I was just now truly enjoying new beginnings.

My husband and I went to the surgeon together and entered his office. He sat there expressionless, writing something in a patient file. I tentatively greeted him as he motioned silently for us to sit down. With a sober face he stated the "facts".

"You have stage 3C cancer and that means it has spread throughout your abdomen."

"Do you want to see my CAT scans?" I asked meekly, and proceeded to hand them to him.

"I know what they will show." He took the scans, glanced at them and handed them back to me.

"Oh—OK", I said, somewhat befuddled, as I put the films back on the floor.

"So, what is going to happen next week?"

"I will cut you from here (just under my breast bone) to here (almost to my pelvic bone) and I will go around your belly button."

Thank goodness!, I thought. Sure would hate to have my belly button cut in half! I don't usually let anyone touch my belly button. Feels too weird. This all seemed so cold and impersonal, almost as if he were describing to a young fisherman how he would gut a fish.

I asked him, "Doctor, what are my chances of survival?"

"You have a 20 percent chance of survival if all goes well."

"What do you mean if all goes well?"

"I will surgically remove all that I can and then we will start chemotherapy."

"Chemotherapy?" I cried. Surely I hadn't heard him correctly.

"Yes, chemotherapy is your only chance and only if you respond well to it."

"Then, please get this out of me and give me a fighting chance to survive."

"I will do what I can," he stated without smiling. He never smiled once. Lloyd and I both left his office with extremely heavy hearts. *We wait for peace to no avail; for a time of healing, but terror comes instead. (Jeremiah 8:15)* The next hardest part was telling my daughters, Angela and Andraya, along with my mother, Donna, and my father, Luciano (He goes by Louis). Angela was shocked and said, "Mom, you are a strong woman. You can beat this. I'll be there for you." Andraya said, "Mom, you don't deserve this. All of my friends think that you are the coolest mom in the world. I support you in whatever you need to do".

I called the university where I taught to inform them that even though the semester was starting next week I would be unable to teach. I hated to leave them in a bind so suddenly with no time to find another professor, but I saw no other choice. Grading graduate student papers, along with the energy required for planning and lecturing, was just too much to think about. I also had no idea how long it would take to recover from surgery. It's amazing how busy and involved my life was and how difficult it was to bring everything to a grinding halt, like a piece of machinery that suddenly had a crucial gear stripped. My whole life as I knew it came to a complete stop. Lunch with my friends, meeting with clients to show them homes, Friday night margaritas with my husband, getting the car washed, shopping, answering emails, grocery shopping, going to my Italian society meetings, going to church on Sunday, getting my hair cut,....**everything** was at a standstill. *Save me, God, for the waters have reached my neck. I have sunk into the mire of the deep, where there is no foothold. I have gone down to the watery depths; the flood overwhelms me. (Psalm 69:2-3)*

I called Betty, my friend and boss at the university, to tell her the news and the slim chances that the doctor gave me. Something she said really hit me and I will always be grateful to her. She emphatically stated, "Diana, that doctor doesn't even know you. He doesn't know your body. You have a lot going for you. Do not accept what he says." I said, "Betty, you are absolutely right! He DOESN'T know me **or** my body!" For some reason, those statements shook me out of my self-pity mode and into a more hopeful mode. How could someone I'd never met tell me how things were going to be? Only God knows that! *But, rather let him who glories, glory in this, that in his prudence he knows me, knows that I, the Lord, bring about kindness... (Jeremiah 9:23)*

During one of the following days, I went to the bookstore, purchased a blank writing journal entitled *The Wish Journal* (I thought that sounded appropriate). I decided to use it as a diary of all that happened to me, my thoughts, my prayers, and my insights, since I didn't know what lay ahead. Now, I am not a writer, mind you, I am a talker. I could talk your head off. This entire situation, then, offered two challenges. First, I was determined to survive and second, I was going to write about how I successfully accomplished it.

The Chronicles Begin

January 15
Supposedly, they say I have ovarian cancer. It's apparently late in the game. I found all of this out 4 days ago. What a blow to my psyche. I fully plan to be here on this earth quite a while longer and this journal will record how, with the help of family, friends, my husband, and the Lord, that I did it and lived a great life! Read on to discover my secrets as well as my ups and downs and how powerful our thoughts really are. I love my family so dearly and I share this with them so we can celebrate together the victory over disease.

Two days before surgery, the weather turned downright ugly. An ice storm hit and all of the roads were treacherous, at best, but the doctor in charge still wanted me to come in for a colonoscopy. In his pick up truck, Lloyd and I braved the ice, slipping and sliding our way at a snail's pace to the office. This whole situation was getting unbelievable. We live in the south. It only snows about once every 15-20 years. Somebody wake me up! My mother was flying down from Iowa to be with me during and after surgery. I was so thankful to the Lord that my mother was well at the age of 77 and able to travel to be by my side.

January 16
It's cold and dreary, and we've been iced in all day, but I carry sunshine in my heart. I love and know that I am loved, so it is never dreary inside. My friends are calling and I thank them for it. I already feel like a survivor. I have to drink some gross phosphate so it will "clean me out" for the colonoscopy.

I received a call from a friend who wants to buy a house.

Good thing my husband can take over. Oh, Lord, help me through this as only you can. I love you and trust you Jesus. Amen

January 17
I tried to be brave and have the colonoscopy with no sedation but the pain was too great so I gave in and let them give me anesthesia to put me in the twilight zone. The doctor said the inside of the colon looks clear! Thank you, Jesus! It's the first good news. I believe, oh Lord, in your mercy and goodness.

Angela and her husband, Dustin, came to spend the night. It is wonderful to see them. Supportive family is your life-blood. I cherish them always. I am ready to win with your help, oh Lord. You are my rock and my salvation. My hope is in YOU. Amen

What was I thinking to try and have this colonoscopy without anesthesia? I think I wanted to be fully awake and see for myself what might be present in the colon. It was the part of me that wants to be in control of my life. I felt it was humiliating to ask for medication. I didn't like people "doing things" to my body and felt powerless. When the probing camera hit a bend in my colon, the pain was just too much for me. I surrendered. With the good news from the internist, maybe it wasn't as bad as they were telling me. The surgery would be in two days. In the meantime, my abdomen kept swelling and was really getting uncomfortable. What was in there anyway? I wanted to have some magic camera to see inside of myself. Whatever it was, it had to go. It could not be part of me any longer. *Give heed to the voice of my cry, my King and my God, for to You I will pray. (Psalm 5:2)*

Surgery and the Aftermath

January 19 dawned as another cold, miserable, icy day. Lloyd and I headed to the hospital early in the morning. I hated getting up so darned early with a hungry belly just to go somewhere and be put back to sleep again. By now, my abdomen had swollen so badly that I could not even get my largest pants zipped up halfway. It was so embarrassing and I waddled like a pregnant woman. Thank goodness for those gigantic hospital gowns. They can hide a multitude of things, at least in the FRONT which was right where I needed it.

I waited patiently on the gurney outside the surgery *suite* (as they call it). I would rather have been enjoying a *suite* in a vacation condo somewhere. The smell of the hospital was actually a comfortably familiar scent since I had worked in a hospital as a medical laboratory scientist for a few years right after college. So, at least I didn't have a fear of hospitals like some people do. The hospital was abuzz with different members of the surgery staff hustling to and fro. The anesthesiologist came in and asked me if I was allergic to a bunch of things and told me what sleepy-time drugs they were going to give me. It is so nice of them to explain all of this even though they can tell that you have no clue about these drugs, with complicated names, that they mention so casually. Then the surgery nurse came in and asked me the same allergy questions again. I wanted to say that I was allergic to tumors so could they please hurry and get any out of me. But, I kept my tongue in check which was getting pretty thick from the IV relaxation drugs they had given me. My mother had arrived the night before, so she, my daughters, and husband were all in the surgery waiting room. The magic hour had arrived and they wheeled me into surgery. *Let your hand be with me, and keep me from harm so that I shall be free from pain. (I Chronicles 4:10)*

Right before surgery, the laboratory performed a cancer cell count from my blood to get some idea of how bad the cancer was. This test is called a CA-125. (They have different ones for different types of cancer.) The normal cell count (since supposedly we all have some cancer cells) was 21. Therefore, the lower it is, the better. My count was around 1,500.

The surgery lasted approximately 3 hours. After going inside my abdomen, the doctor had to remove the ovaries, fallopian tubes, and many parts of my large intestine. Even though the cancer was not inside the colon, apparently, it had attached itself to several places on the outside of the colon. About half way through the surgery, the doctor called the waiting room and told my husband that they had removed so many parts of the colon that I would probably need a colostomy bag. Although he was disappointed, Lloyd told him to do whatever he needed to do to give me a chance at survival. The moment Lloyd got off the phone with the doctor, my whole family prayed earnestly to the Lord to spare me from having a colostomy bag to deal with, in addition to what was to come. The surgeon also cauterized (burned off) several tumors on my liver, bladder, and other organs, including my diaphragm. When the surgery was over, the doctor came out and talked to the family. He informed them that, miraculously, they were able to piece the parts of my large intestine together with lots of stitches and did not have to put in a colostomy bag after all. He said that they had removed about 99% of the tumors. My family rejoiced and thanked the Lord for hearing and answering their prayers. I was already receiving the benefit from the spiritual realm. He also informed them that they had removed almost a gallon of fluid and at least 8 pounds of tumors. No wonder I weighed so much!

Pain and lots of pain. That is all I remember for the few moments of awakening from that day, but I was so thankful that I had survived! I had a fear, going into surgery, of never waking up again. I vaguely saw Lloyd's face in a fog in the recovery room and said to him in my hoarse whispery voice, "It hurts so badly." Lloyd said they had some sort of 'warming gown' wrapped around me hooked up to a machine. This machine would pump warm air all around me. My body temperature hovered around 94 degrees. He also revealed to me later that the nurse told him that he had to leave because they were going to give me a good dose of morphine.

Yet if I speak, my pain is not relieved; and if I refrain, it does not go away. Surely, O God, you have worn me out... (Job 16:6-7) When I gained some consciousness, I realized that there were at least four tubes coming into and out of me.

For example, I felt an irritation itch in my neck and when I tried to scratch it, was somewhat horrified to discover that they had put an IV line in my jugular vein! It was taped heavily to my neck, and hooked up to a thick, white, pasty substance that was to be my food for the next few weeks. This made a stomach feeding tube, which they had also inserted into me during surgery, look like child's play. All during the day and night, the alarm for that jugular IV sounded off and on because the feeding IV line continuously became clogged. How could anyone possibly rest with a beeping alarm going off constantly, and the nurses coming in and trying various things to unclog it? And it was inside of a large vital vein going directly to my heart! The stomach tube was not comfortable and neither was the urinary catheter. I tried rolling over with all of those things attached....impossible.

There was another line hooked up to a morphine drip. That line I liked pretty well with its 'thumb button' I got to push whenever I needed a dose. One day when I was in a great amount of pain, I kept pushing that button on the machine, waiting for the morphine to kick in. When the nurse entered to check my neck IV, I asked, "Why isn't this morphine working? I've pushed this button about 10 times!" She had an amused look on her face and stated, "It only allows you to get a dose every 6 minutes. You can keep pushing that button until you get 'video game thumb' and nothing is going to happen until 6 minutes have gone by. Doctor's orders." Shoot! They had fooled me! I had been so happy thinking I could have that 'good feeling juice' anytime I wanted! Because I stayed on my back most of the time in the bed, my back became irritated from sweat. Due to the antibiotics they were giving me, I got a yeast infection on my back and in my mouth (called thrush). Was I having fun yet?

The next few days are gone from memory until much later when the hospital staff was forcing me to get out of bed and walk. I am convinced that no one gets any rest in a hospital—not the staff and not the patients. After getting awakened every couple of hours for something different: blood work, respiratory therapy, temperature and blood pressure checks, that annoying alarm going off, and so on, I was totally exhausted. I practically begged to just be left alone. What did I think this was? A hotel with a "do not disturb" sign? No such luck. *Come to me all you who are weary and burdened, and I will give you rest. Take my yoke upon you and learn from me, for I am gentle and humble in heart, and you will find rest for your souls. (Matthew 11:28-29)* I badly needed complete rest. In looking back, I should have prayed and asked the Lord to help me with finding rest.

> January 24
> Cold and dreary day…I have been to hell and back. (Actually, still working my way out of the darkness.) The pain from the surgery was <u>unbelievable</u> and the lack of sleep discouraging. I so badly need uninterrupted sleep and rest. I thank the Lord that every day it is beginning to lessen. Now, I am waiting for my re-sectioned large intestine to start passing gas. I guess that is how they determine whether or not it is working. I just hope it doesn't start doing that when I have visitors. I feel my recovery beginning to happen and I am visualizing myself and my family taking a trip to Italy. I plan to be healthier than before and be a new person.
>
> I went for a walk down the corridor with mom and when we returned, the doctor was lying on the bed, hands behind his head, with feet crossed. He said, "I passed gas today, did you?" I laughed so much. And I blessed him. He had a sense of humor after all.
>
> Several friends have stopped by and my mother has been here every day. Thank you, Lord, for family and friends.

Ha! I could still think and I could still pray. I talked quite a bit to God in that hospital room. When I felt pain, when I couldn't sleep, when I was alone, or for any reason, I told God everything and thanked him for the success of my surgery. I am so thankful it was a private room since I talked out loud at times. Every day, I took a walk and pushed myself to walk just a little farther down the hospital hallway, with my pole that held the multiple tubes, bags, and a monitor. It was extremely exhausting. My mother, among many other things, washed my back as I stood unsteadily in the shower each day, while holding the tubes out of the way. Then, she'd help me dry off and put on a new hospital gown (I still hate those things). Now, that is truly someone who loves you. I was so grateful for her presence that some days, I would cry. Lloyd visited too, but had a full time job and all of the household matters to continue, so kept his visits short. I could tell he just didn't feel comfortable hanging around a hospital room.

Angela and Dustin, Andraya and fiancé Derek, as well as many friends came to visit me and were so encouraging. Even the flowers they brought were a way of feeling like I had a bit of spring and sunshine in the room with me, despite the weather outside (which was still extremely cold and wintry). Matt Kuglics, a soldier stationed here, who was one of my clients that I viewed like a son, came to visit in between Iraq assignments and defending our country. Maggie, my friend with her own cancer issues, visited and brought food for my family. Everyone was so thoughtful. I could never repay all of the kindness. *But the fruit of the Spirit is love, joy, peace, patience, kindness, goodness, faithfulness, gentleness, and self-control. Against such things, there is no law. (Galatians 5:22-23)*

The doctor ordered another CA-125 and the number now stood at 133. What a drastic improvement! It was very encouraging. Maybe now, my body could somehow begin to rid itself of these unwelcome cells. I asked for some paper and tape from the nurses and hung up a sign on the wall that I could see every time I opened my eyes. On it I wrote, "I am in perfect continual health." I focused on that one statement and prayed.

What I did not know was that every night, my family gathered at our house and formed a prayer circle to pray for me, thinking positive, healing thoughts. This brought them closer together. There had never been a time that all of them had prayed together. That, in itself, was a beautiful manifestation of the power of the Holy Spirit. Most times, events like these are not about us. They are about other people. All the people around you are being affected in some way. Hard to believe, but in retrospect, I'm beginning to understand.

January 28
A sunny day! Oh, as I lay looking out of the hospital window, I wished that I could feel the sunshine on my face! I long for the simple things. I saw a single star outside my hospital room window and it carries my wish to the Lord. Starlight, star bright, I wish for...Total healing and cure. It's coming—I believe it.

They gave me a dose of Milk of Magnesia last night to "get things moving" in my poor stitched up bowel. It worked too well. Diarrhea is too nice of a word. I was up almost all night back and forth to the bathroom, tiredly dragging my tubes and bags with me. All I can say is that they must have used tons of iodine for surgery because I was full of it! It's too gross to describe the rest—even for a personal diary.

January 29
Good morning, Lord! I have just realized that all that I have to do every morning is arise! That is all! The rest is up to my God and Lord to direct as he wishes. So, today is here and I'm ready. The doctor said I can try solid foods.

I had 2 wonderful meals! I don't even care that it was hospital food. It wasn't through a stomach tube. Hallelujah! I feel great! (As good as I can anyway!) So many people have come by to visit. I love them all.

The only thought running through my head, after 10 days, was what most people desire as soon as they find themselves in the hospital; "When can I go home?" I asked it of the doctor, the nurses, and the Lord. Each day was slow improvement—less morphine needed, more ability to walk almost upright, less tired than the day before, and able to do more for myself. Finally, the day arrived to depart, when all tubes and the 44 metal staples were removed.

"Good morning," said the doctor as he entered with a towel over his arm (like a waiter about to serve a bottle of champagne) and something that resembled a pair of pliers.

"Good morning, doctor. I'm ready to go home so what do we have to do?"

"And how are you doing this morning?" he asked, as he got the "pliers" ready.

"I'm doing fine." I said while he pulled out the staples one by one and placed them in a tray. It felt like a mild bee sting each time.

"And what do you want to do when you get home?" he asked innocently.

"Well, first I want to— Ouch! That hurt so much!" I shrieked. I felt a sharp pain at the same time I saw, in front of my face, the now exposed stomach tube he had just yanked out of me, dripping onto the towel the contents of the breakfast I had eaten. That was enough to take away my good mood at going home...almost. A few cuss words came to mind, but I try to be a good Christian.

"That was easy." he stated calmly.

"You could have warned me." I said forlornly as I looked at a gaping hole into my stomach. "Aren't you going to stitch it up or anything?"

"Nope."

The nurse standing nearby said, "I'm going to put a bandage on the wound."

"Is that all you are going to do?"

"Yes, just keep it covered. It might leak for a little while, but eventually it will seal up on its own".

"Are you sure?" I asked. Just what I needed—a gaping hole in my midsection.

"Absolutely. Just change the dressings when you shower. And now I'm going to need you to lie perfectly still because I'm going to remove the IV line from your neck."

"Please be gentle. I'm still hurting from the stomach tube getting yanked so rudely out of me."

"Don't worry. Just relax. I will do this as gently as I can." She peeled all the tape off my neck, ever so gingerly.

"Good so far, but I'm trying to remain calm."

"It's going well. Now, don't freak out when I remove the IV line because the tube is about nine inches into your jugular vein—almost into your heart."

"I'm glad I didn't know that all this time!" What a strange sensation that was as the tube seemed to crawl slowly up my neck.

"Ah, here it is," she stated while she showed it to me.

"Whoa! That whole thing was in me?"

"It sure was. I'm going to stand here and keep pressure on the vein for about 30 minutes." I hoped she wouldn't get tired.

After we made small talk for a very long 30 minutes and I realized that I was still breathing, intact, and not bleeding anywhere, she put a bandage on my neck and said, "You must continue to lie down for at least an hour and I'll be in periodically to check on you." Oh, glory day! No more incessant beeping from the alarm for a clogged IV feeding line. Freedom from the tubes! "Isn't the body remarkable?" I thought as I lay there waiting patiently for the neck wound to "seal itself". If that is the case, how had my body initially betrayed me? How had I betrayed it? How could this be changed?

The nurse re-entered the room. "Let me look—yes—it looks good. You can get up now and I'll call patient services to bring you a wheelchair for the ride downstairs."

"That will be great—my husband's on his way."

"Good. Well, I guess we'll see you again in about 6 months."

"Why are you going to see me in about 6 months?" I asked with a puzzled look on my face.

"Why, for your second-look surgery."

"Second-look surgery? WHAT is THAT?" I asked, my voice pitch rising with alarm.

"After chemotherapy and any other treatments, the doctor usually repeats the same surgery to make sure there is no cancer hiding in there."

"Oh, I see," was all I could dumbly say. NO way. No way am I doing this again. One surgery was bad enough but two surgeries? The same 15-20 inch cut? The same excruciating pain? No way. Right now, I just wanted to get home.

> January 30
> I'm home! Oh, my Lord. It feels so good to be in my own home, my own bathroom, and my own bed, with no one waking me up constantly. Hallelujah! I can go to the restroom without an IV pole and tubes! Oh, the <u>simple</u> things I have missed. And I've missed snuggling with my husband. He has been so supportive. The pain is still here from the surgery but getting less every day. The wounds from my stomach tube, IV's, and staples are improving too. Thank you Jesus. I trust you.

The next several days and nights were tough. I was unable to sleep through the night. I found myself sitting up in a lounge chair for part of the night, lying on the floor, and trying the couch, to find a comfortable position. My bowels were still not working properly, there was still pain, and I visited the restroom at least 20 times a day. I never knew when the urge would hit, so I was afraid to go anywhere where there wasn't a restroom for longer than 10 minutes. I longed for the day when this would subside and yet wondered if it ever would. I felt pain and fear. My bladder hurt. It was painful to urinate. During the cold days, I put on my coat and gloves, and took a very short walk. My mom walked too, but I could tell that she was cold. She stoically braved the chill to encourage me. I allowed my body to begin healing, to receive fresh air (even cold air), sunshine, and some exercise. What lay ahead of me? Could I be strong?

During the hospitalization, my daughters had already started reading books on changing one's eating habits to restore health. They read that sugar fed cancer, that salt upset the potassium/sodium balance, and that strong antioxidants were needed. So, they went through my pantry, cupboards, and refrigerator and tossed out ANYTHING that had sugar or salt (which was one-half of my diet!). They purchased antioxidant drinks, immune boosting supplements, and anything else that they thought might be helpful. I truly believe that this was how they dealt with the shock and anger of the situation. Even my favorite chocolate was gone, as well as my chocolate chip pieces for baking! It especially upset me that they tossed out the popcorn salt I had searched for and finally found. They were serious! In retrospect, I owe them deep gratitude for the love they exhibited.

My mother stayed another two weeks to help out and was invaluable. She helped with meals and many people brought food. Of course, some people brought sweets, which I needed to avoid, and I asked them not to bring any more. That was tough. I didn't want to seem ungrateful but my LIFE was at stake here. My dad stayed in Iowa with my handicapped brother. I talked with him on the phone and felt his love also. Love is a powerful thing.

Even though it was still bitter cold outside, I donned my winter coat and my mom and I took another walk for as far as I could make it. As I moved, my lungs felt like they were on fire, my footsteps felt heavy, my chest heaved, I felt like I couldn't get enough oxygen, but each day, we went a little further. Each day, it got a little easier. I thanked God for what I could do and looked forward to steady improvement. Eventually, mom had to get back home. I missed her terribly, but knew she needed to be back with my dad and brother. It's always good to get back home—I had just experienced that feeling.

Back to the Doctor

It was now the first week in February and time to go to the gynecological oncologist (who had performed the surgery) for a check up, although I was still somewhat weakened from surgery and didn't feel quite well enough yet. Abdominal discomfort remained and I wasn't sleeping comfortably. The bowels were a little more under control with only 10 visits to the restroom a day now. It still didn't feel right to urinate. What had he done to my bladder? The surgeon was such a serious looking and sounding fellow. That alone was enough to make me afraid. After our greetings, he began talking about next steps.

"Doctor, what happened to my bladder? Why does it bother me so much?"

"I really had to scrape it to get the cancer off of the outside."

"No wonder it hurts."

"I think you are healed enough to start chemotherapy." He stated.

"But, doctor, I don't want chemotherapy. I've heard about all of the horrible things it does." I was afraid of even the word, let alone the effects.

"You need to stop listening to people about that."

"But they are people who have experienced it."

He said, "You need to be more afraid of the cancer than the chemotherapy." I disagreed, but had no information that would allow me to argue the point. After all, who studies up on cancer and treatments unless they have it or someone they love has it?

I asked him, "Aren't there any other choices? What about immunotherapy?" (I'd at least heard the word somewhere.)

"None of those other ideas are proven. Chemotherapy is your best chance." He very casually stated, "You will lose your hair, but it will grow back again." Did he realize what he was saying to me? I am half Italian! I've always had gloriously thick dark Italian hair. People have been envious of my head of hair and now here he was, flippantly informing me that it would be gone soon. Why should it be this way? What type of "medicine" kills your hair? Of all times to have to lose my hair, this was the worst. After all, it was the middle of winter! Did I have to accept this? It seemed like my only choice.

"OK then, if you feel that this is what is best for me."

"Fine, we'll start chemotherapy next week." He called for his nurse while he wrote out the "prescription." His nurse appeared and, after introductions, led me down the hall.

"Here is the room where we give the medication." she said while showing me the "chemotherapy room". She explained the process to me and said that I would be coming every three weeks for a treatment. Sitting or lying on the beds were 5 or 6 women, most with no hair and scarves on their heads, receiving the chemical chosen for them by the doctor. They were reading, watching television, or lying down. Dejected, scared, and still in disbelief, I left his office for home.

During the next few days, my daughters both implored me not to take the chemotherapy. Angela said, "Mom, that stuff is nothing but pure poison. It totally destroys the body and the immune system. There are other ways."

"But, Angela, I don't KNOW any other way. I feel lost and afraid."

"Check with other people, mom. Don't give in to this!"

"I don't think I have any other choice! I'm going to try the chemotherapy."

Andraya said that she had a friend who was doing well and completely taking care of himself after a serious diagnosis of cancer by taking supplements and other things he had researched on the internet. She also encouraged me to explore other avenues.

Gaitano, my friend from the Italian organization I belong to, called me several times and said, "Diana, please don't take the chemotherapy. I met someone who went to a holistic clinic here, was cured of cancer, and is doing great today. You ought to give the clinic a call."

"Thanks, Tom (his nickname), but I've already scheduled chemo to start next week." Why did I not believe that the same holistic cure could happen to me? Did she have the same diagnosis? Because if she didn't, there was no way I would believe in that type of treatment. I know better now, but when I first was diagnosed, I thought each type of cancer was unique. Cancer is cancer. It only differs slightly according to which organ is involved.

"Do you know what she had, Tom? Could I call and talk to her?"

"I'll get her number and call you back."

"Thanks, I appreciate that." A few minutes later, he called with her number.

I called feeling very apprehensive. Her husband answered and said she was in the shower. He asked who I was and what I wanted. I awkwardly explained. He said she'd return my call. She never did and I didn't call back.

Tom kept insisting that I at least call the Holistic Health Care Center in Boerne (pronounced like the name Bernie), Texas, to discover what they had to offer. (Boerne is just outside San Antonio.) Reluctantly, I called and asked them to send me some information. This was all so confusing and overwhelming. What was I to do? I didn't want the chemotherapy, but that is all I'd heard about and I trusted the doctor, at least somewhat. All I could do now was pray and wait.

February 10

Chemo starts next week. I am brave. I will have minimal side effects. Oh, Holy Spirit, come and dwell within me and fill me with your truth.

We bought a juicer, but I don't know if I can really get into that. Betty M, my friend from the University where I was teaching and her husband, Bruce, brought me a portable CD/ cassette player to listen to positive tapes. I am lost, Lord, but I thank you, for all you have brought into my life. Amen

I inundated myself with ANY sources of hope, including the Bible, positive tapes, books of hope, and movies. Whenever people called and asked what they could do, I told them, "Bring me anything that speaks of hope, healing, and health." I was surrounded by resources with the Lord bringing me more everyday. Angela gave me a set of breathing tapes because cancer does not like oxygen. I decided that my body was going to become a new place, one that did not harbor or welcome anything that shouldn't be there. I asked the Lord to bring me whatever it would take to achieve that end.

February 11

My friend Diana came over today. Together, we prayed and visualized my total health with perfectly functioning organs and cells. She directed me to take a reclining position on the sofa and told me we were going to talk to the cancer cells. We asked them what it would take to make them go away. The answer was most interesting. The cancer cells are not happy because I am changing the environment of my body and mind. My body is becoming extremely unwelcoming to them so they are going to leave. I imagined myself on a beach, marveling how wonderful it felt to be totally healthy. I am full of the Lord's white light. Oh, Lord, I am so grateful to you for all of these healing resources. Thank you Lord. Amen.

Now, I felt ready to face anything! My spirits were lifted and I was sure that this whole thing would be no problem. My body was strong and I would surprise them all. How bad could this chemotherapy stuff be? I could certainly overcome whatever harmful effect it had on me as long as it got rid of those nasty cancer cells.

As soon as I told people about the cancer diagnosis, I heard the horror stories about chemotherapy. They said it made one ill, food didn't taste good *if* you could keep it down, you got weak and constantly tired, and an entire host of bad effects—too numerous to mention. I listened to them, but couldn't really absorb what it meant for me. The night before my first treatment, Lloyd took me to an Italian restaurant. As the waitress greeted us she casually asked, "Is this a special occasion?" I guess it was, but not in the way she expected. I answered, "Well, tomorrow I will receive my first chemotherapy treatment and tonight I am going to eat like a queen! We'll start with a glass of wine please." With a stunned look and unable to find the words to reply, she hurried off to get the wine. She came back with the bottle and two glasses and filled them almost to overflowing. What a tremendous meal. It's strange how we take eating for granted until it is not an ordinary normal event. It was like eating my last meal before facing the executioner. I made sure that I savored the taste of every bite, for who knew what tomorrow would bring.

Heavenly Pearls of Wisdom

Listen to your body. You have lived with it. You KNOW when something isn't right. Pursue it at all costs and don't let anyone downplay any symptoms.

Do not panic. Many people panic when given a serious diagnosis and the mind runs amuck with chaos and confusion.

Pray and step back. Pray as long as it takes to get calm and/or receive answers and guidance.

Call only a few of your trusted relatives and friends. Many others will only add to your panic, confusion, and fear.

Calmly search for surgeons, healers, herbalists, etc. You want an entire balanced team working with you and for you.

2
Into the Darkness

The next day, Thursday, dawned wintry cold but not as dreary. Lloyd took me to chemo the first time because I didn't know what to expect. I needed him there to hold my hand and provide emotional support. My friends told me to bring books to read and puzzles to do along with some food to eat to pass the time while getting the chemotherapy treatment. I wore a short sleeved t-shirt and sweatpants with tennis shoes to be comfortable. I brought my "bag of goodies", including my own pillow. I tried to think of this as a just another experience. I actually felt pretty healthy.

Traditional Treatment Begins

We arrived at the doctor's chemotherapy center containing six hospital beds with pretty quilts on them. Four were empty so far.

"Good morning, Diana," said the nurse. "Why don't you select an empty bed and make yourself comfortable." Was she serious? How can someone who is about to get some chemical in their veins get comfortable?

"Nurse, I am very frightened and nervous about all of this."

"Don't worry. We are going to take good care of you. First, we are going to take a look at your veins," she stated as she put a tourniquet on my arm and waited. Thank goodness, I inherited good veins, nice and firm, and near the surface.

"Would it be all right to use a vein in my hand? Since I'm going to be coming every three weeks, I don't want to wear out the big arm veins." (I'd seen enough of that in my days as a medical laboratory scientist.)

"Well, let's see. Yes, you can use a hand vein, but it might be more uncomfortable for you." (I should have known what that meant—it meant painful.) She put the tourniquet around my wrist, plumped up the vein and inserted the needle. Yikes! What was I thinking? That smarted. She promptly taped the needle in place on the back of my hand.

"First, I'm going to hook up an intravenous line with some saline solution to make sure that the line is working."

"OK, how long will that take?"

"Just a few minutes," she stated. My heart was already pounding with fear as the minutes ticked by slowly. I didn't like it already.

"Now, I'm going to give you something to relax," she soothingly said as she injected a syringe full of something into the IV line. Now that part I liked.

"I feel like I've just had two glasses of wine. Well, so far this is not bad and I feel pretty good." She smiled.

"This is an anti-nausea medication," she said as she switched out the saline bag for a smaller one.

"How long does <u>that</u> one take?"

"Usually about 15 minutes and I'll be nearby if you need me." Time passed slowly and my hand was beginning to sting at the site of the IV. Once again, she was at my side.

"Ok, I'm going to start the chemo now." I watched apprehensively as she replaced the bag with another big one. "But, I am only going to start with two drops into the line." And then the moment of truth came. I watched as she cautiously opened the valve and let two drops into the line. The reaction was immediate.

"Oh, my God! It hurts so bad!" I gasped. My entire insides felt as if someone had twisted them into a knot. "I feel like my head is on fire too!" My face became extremely red and my head and scalp felt torched afire with gasoline.

"Try to stay calm."

"I can't! My chest is tightening! I can hardly breathe!" I thought I was having a heart attack, had been stabbed with a knife, and been torched, all at one time.

"Ok, I'm going to help you. Just hold on."

"Please hurry! I can't take the pain!" I thought I was dying. The pain was excruciating. The nurse quickly ran over to her emergency cabinet and ran back with a syringe full of epinephrine. She swiftly injected it into my IV line.

"There now, it will get better soon."

"I still feel horrible!" I said as I gasped for breath.

"You had a reaction to the drug and we'll have to try a different one. At least 10% of people react to Taxol™." She took my blood pressure and it was 200 over 130 which is way above normal. My pulse still raced at over 100. What had this "medicine" done to me? What sort of cruelty was this? Oh, why did I choose this and how could I get out of it? I just wanted to go home.

"Why didn't you tell me this could happen?" I asked, incredulous.

"Because you would have been more frightened, possibly for nothing. Just breathe deeply while I go talk to the doctor." She and the doctor consulted while Lloyd tried to calm me and himself down.

Thirty minutes later she said, "Well, we're going to give you a drug called Gemsar™. So the good news is that you won't lose your hair and not one of our patients has had a reaction to this one." By this time I think Lloyd had seen enough to horrify him, but he stayed with me.

"Are you sure this drug will not do to me what the last one did?" I asked shakily.

"You'll be fine. Everyone does well on this. You'll have to come in every week with this drug, instead of every 3 weeks." She then hooked up the new bag and let it begin to slowly drip into my veins. This was accompanied by a burning and stinging sensation in my entire arm.

"My hand is really burning! Is there anything you can do?"

"Unfortunately, that happens with this drug. I'll bring something for you in just a minute." She brought warm towels to put on my hand and arm. She checked with me a few minutes later. "How is your hand doing?"

"It feels a little bit better. I'll be glad when this is over." The bag drained ever so slowly. My bowels still weren't back to normal so I had to get up several times during treatment to use the restroom. I dragged my pole with IV to the restroom (which was very small and required ingenious maneuvering) each time. This in itself was exhausting, since I did not want to have any "accidents" on the bedding.

Finally, the bag emptied. "Time to remove your IV line," said the nurse while she unhooked everything, removing the tape and needle. So much for reading, working puzzles, and eating. This experience had been worse than a trip to a bad hotel. My hand and arm were still stinging. When would that go away? Before I left, the nurse gave me two slips of paper. "Here are prescriptions for nausea. Start taking them tomorrow evening (Friday) because you might feel some discomfort on Saturday. We'll see you next week at the same time." Supposedly, I had two days before the "discomfort" hit. Again, the word "discomfort" did not prepare me for what was to come.

By the next day, Friday, I awakened with excruciating stomach pain and nausea. I was sure that my insides had twisted themselves up into a rebellious knot. I would have been happy with just "discomfort". And I had not taken the anti-nausea medicine because I wasn't supposed to take it until that evening. The entire day, I literally crawled around on the floor and prayed for relief. Try to eat?

Forget it! I knew I needed nourishment, but my stomach wasn't interested. What had they done to my body? This seemed worse than any diagnosis or disease. *I am withered, dried up like grass, too wasted to eat my food. Lord, hear my prayer; let my cry come to you. Do not hide your face from me now that I am in distress. Turn your ear to me; when I call, answer me quickly. (Psalm 102: 5, 2-3)*

In seven days, I was going to get more of this stuff! O, Lord, give me strength. Mercifully, I slept on and off the better part of the next day. But, each time I awakened, the nausea was there to greet me. Maybe sleeping through all of this was the answer. Yeah. Right. Doing any real estate or even taking care of household chores was impossible. That took energy. I owe a large measure of gratitude to my housecleaning person and friend, Lynn. She kept the house clean, made me smoothies, and asked how she could help. How do people survive this? How do they have the will to do so—especially if they don't have a support system?

> February 18
> Well, after the bad reaction to Taxol™, at least I don't lose my hair. I've had to deal with nausea for the past 3 days and one day of sleeping in addition. Oh, I hope that I will be able to get these things under control—figure out what needs to be done—what I can eat—I don't want to lose any more weight—I want to maintain and get healthy. I am at 116 pounds. I weighed that when I was 24. I must help my immune system. Oh, Lord, I ask you for the answers. I know they are there. This is, after all, my WELLNESS journal. I AM getting well. The cancer cells are not welcome and they can leave NOW, all of them. May God bless Lloyd and my support systems, to keep them strong. I know it is hard on the care givers and I pray for all care givers.

The following days I felt better, but queasiness and fatigue persisted. To me, this was much worse than the recovery from surgery. At least after surgery, I knew that I was slowly improving every day. With this treatment, I didn't know what each new day would be like. Every day brought nausea and not much energy, but I managed to eat some things that tasted good (like mashed potatoes) and keep them down. I became increasingly upset because I knew deep in my core that my body needed extra nutrition to overcome the situation yet, most foods, especially anything with protein in it, were unappealing to me. Sure would have liked a candy bar or a milk shake.

The Second Treatment

The day before my next treatment, I actually ate a fast food sandwich! Thank you Lord! It tasted good and I did a little shopping. Very therapeutic. I didn't go out for too long since my bowels still acted up. Before my second treatment, the doctor's office said to go to the lab and get blood work done to see how the counts for my white cells (the ones that fight infection), red cells (the ones that carry oxygen) and my platelets (the ones responsible for blood clotting) were doing. Dutifully, I complied and then received my second treatment of chemotherapy. I drove unaccompanied this time because I didn't want to subject Lloyd, nor anyone else, to that again. Following the session, I took the anti-nausea medicine that same night. The next day, I felt nauseated but not like the intense pain of the first treatment. Maybe I could suffer through this after all with ONLY 16 more treatments left. *Out of the depths I call to you, Lord; Lord, hear my cry! May your ears be attentive. (Psalm 130:1)*

> February 19
> Well, my friends say that this experience is a journey. If so, what kind of journey am I really on? Where am I going? What am I supposed to learn from this? — To spend more time with God?— To love life more than I already do?— To deeply appreciate all of the people in my life? I await the insights because so far all it does is HURT!

The Third Treatment

The time arrived for my third treatment a week later. Friends offered to take me to treatment and I decided that I needed the moral support. My friend Mary Nell picked me up in her car and accompanied me. As I wearily entered the therapy area, the nurse immediately informed me that she had received the results of my laboratory tests. My counts were very low and she gave me two shots, one to boost up my white cells, and one to boost up my red cells. I asked her what the possible side effects were. She said that my joints and muscles might ache and I might get a headache. Just what I needed—a headache and achy joints on top of the nausea.

In spite of all of the low counts, they gave me yet ANOTHER dose of chemotherapy. No wonder I was tired! However, the doctor said that he was going to lower the dose because it was too strong. Good grief! How much were they giving me? I had no idea of the dosage, nor what that dosage meant. At least with a prescription drug in a bottle, I knew how many milligrams I was getting. With chemotherapy, I was clueless! And if I asked for a lower dosage, how would I know if they actually gave me a lower dose?

The only advice was not to be around crowds of people or I might get an infection. This was not healing as I envisioned it. I spent the next two days in bed or on the couch, weak, tired, and nauseated. Inexplicably, all I wanted to watch on television was the cooking channel. How I missed enjoying good food. Even though I had no appetite, I ate because I knew it was important to do so. At least I could eat egg salad. *Have pity on me, Lord, for I am weak; heal me, Lord, for my bones are trembling. (Psalm 6:3)*

I received a statement from the doctor for the insurance company and each chemotherapy treatment was $11,000! And each shot was $6,000! This absolutely floored me. The drug companies are definitely making money and somebody is making lots of money off of the insurance companies and patients. I believed that the drug companies should be paying me for voluntarily allowing them to destroy my body.

February 22

My white blood count went down very low, so I will not get chemo next week. I have a mixed set of feelings—not happy about the white cell count but glad not to get chemo. The white blood count is normally 4-10 and my count was 2.3.

I arose this morning and thanked Jesus for the day before and told him that I hoped I had accomplished whatever was his purpose for me. I received this as a reply: **"It is not always about my purpose. Do you not remember that I have given you all on the earth to enjoy and that I made man lord over all creatures on earth?"** That was the first time I had heard him speak to me in the last several months. I was beginning to think the experience with my cat never happened. I think the message is this—be happy, find joy in the things given to us on earth, and be at peace. I guess one thing is to STOP worrying about what my purpose is. I hope I am serving you in some way. Good advice, Jesus. Thanks and praise to you. Amen.

Is That YOU God?

Was I really receiving thoughts or words from the Lord? Where else would they be coming from? *For God does speak, perhaps once, or even twice, though one perceive it not. (Job 33:14)* The words I heard certainly encouraged me. The Lord had been silent since the healing of my cat Snickers (see Prologue for explanation). Could I trust that these thoughts were Him speaking to me again? I struggled with what to believe and absolutely no one could help me with this. The one Being who could help me was the very one that I doubted really spoke to ordinary people. I thought that He only spoke to Moses, Abraham, and the prophets, and yet, here I was getting very clear words in my head. Is this what the Bible meant when it said *He who has ears to hear, let him hear! (Matthew 13:9)*? If I told anyone, they would think it was an effect of the chemotherapy acting upon my brain. Everybody told me that you get chemo brain when on treatment. Even though I doubted, I was going to take in and enjoy what I was "hearing".

Some people receive messages in prophetic dreams, just like Mary's husband Joseph did. Remember, he wasn't even married to Mary yet, but was already thinking about divorcing her quietly because she was carrying Jesus in her womb. *Such was his intention when, behold, an angel of the Lord appeared to him in a dream and said, 'Joseph, son of David, do no be afraid to take Mary your wife into your home. For it is through the Holy Spirit that this child has been conceived in her.' (Matthew 1:20)* Job also speaks concerning how God communicates when he says, *In a dream, in a vision of the night, (when deep sleep falls upon men) as they slumber in their beds, it is then he opens the ears of men... (Job 33:15)* But, personally, many of my dreams are crazy and don't make much sense. They definitely are not clear messages from angels. At times, I ask the Lord if there is any meaning to them. God speaks to each person in his own way.

Someone asked me, "What is it like when the Lord speaks to you? Do you hear your own voice? Do you hear a booming voice? A deep voice? What is it actually like?" For me, it is simply what I call a "break through thought". I might be in the middle of doing something ordinary and all of a sudden a gentle, sometimes repetitive thought comes into my head. It shakes me out of thinking about whatever I had going on. It "breaks through," similar to when one is listening to a radio station and all of a sudden, a severe weather alert comes on. That definitely gets our attention, because it is so totally different from the music that we were just listening to. That is how God speaks to me. *Listen to my voice; then I will be your God and you shall be my people. (Jeremiah 7:23)*

Back to Chemotherapy

The problem with skipping a chemotherapy session is that it stretches out the length of time for the treatments. I was expected to complete the same number of treatments, no matter how long it took or what it did to me in the process. My friend and Avon lady, Pam, was diagnosed with breast cancer 4 months prior and told she had a 70% chance of survival, if she followed the routine. At least it was better odds than the 20% I'd been given. She was now halfway through with her chemotherapy and her white counts had gotten dangerously low. *Their poison is like the poison of a snake... (Psalm 56:5)* She contracted some sort of infection and fever and ended up in the hospital where she received units of blood and massive doses of antibiotics. In the mean- time, with what little energy I had, I continued to entertain thoughts of alternate ways of healing. Witnessing what my friends were enduring who were further into treatment, made other avenues worthy of investigation.

Another friend from the school district where I had worked, Margaret, offered to take me to my next treatment. It was a day off for the employees. I was amazed that people were lining up to take me. Who would want to do that? What a way to spend her day off. I realized that a friend wasn't just someone you went shopping with or had lunch with. A friend is someone who would take time out of their schedule to do something for you or to talk with you, even when it wasn't convenient for them. I know that I was learning this through the kind actions of others. I prayed to be a better friend to others.

> February 24
> Thank God the nausea was not so bad this week. I was able to eat a chalupa! All things work together for good. Even though I feel so bad, I rejoice at feeling even a little better. Betty came to visit today. Thank you, Lord, for all of the people in my life. Amen.

One of my acquaintances, Mary, brought a friend of hers by the house; Vicki had recovered from stage 4 cancer. She had taken a substance called Essiac Tea that she had obtained from a nearby herbalist. It was developed from an old Canadian Indian root and herb mixture by a nurse with the last name of Caisse. The tea is her name spelled backwards, and it contains 4 basic herbs; sheep sorrel, burdock root, slippery elm, and turkey rhubarb. Rene Caisse had tremendous success with this formula in curing cancer in Canada. How did the doctors and the medical community act when the news of this spread rapidly? They passed a law stating that anyone giving any medicine for cancer not approved by their newly formed cancer commission would be fined for practicing medicine without a license. She had hundreds of letters from cured patients. It made no difference to those in authority.

A drug company enticed her to let them do research on the formula, but would not conduct the research in what she knew was an unbiased manner unless she gave them the exclusive rights to the formula. They wanted to try and isolate one or two compounds from the formula (which is what drug companies do, and in so doing, produce drugs with bad side effects) and market it. This indicated greed and arrogance on their part, so she refused. All she had wanted was to help people get well, especially the poor. The medical establishment eventually caused her to shut down her clinic.

Mary and Vicki asked if I wanted to try some of the Essiac tea they had brewed and I thought, "I am ready to try some other things." I was not ready to give up chemotherapy since my doctor was such an adamant advocate, but possibly take this in addition to it. My mind and heart desperately searched for answers. *You will show me the path to life, abounding joy in your presence, the delights at your right hand forever. (Psalm 16:11)*

February 28
I believe that the Lord is giving me resources such as garlic (a powerful immune booster) and Essiac Tea (a detoxifier). Mary and Vicki brought the tea that Vicky had brewed up and I take 1 oz in the morning and 1 oz in the evening. We prayed together and it is so wonderful. I believe in the resources being given to me. I read a passage written by Mother Teresa

that said we should not fear suffering. She says that one must remember that the passion of Christ ends in the joy of the resurrection and for us, the "resurrection has to come." Oh, Lord Jesus, I await the day of the joy of resurrection and know and believe that it IS coming soon. Amen.

March 2
I actually felt pretty good today—about 85%! Thank you Jesus! So, I did what any woman would do with money, a car, and time. I went shopping! And amazingly, I only had to use the restroom one time! Oh, what a glorious day. I ate lunch outdoors and thanked the Lord for the wonderful feel of sunshine on my back and skin—there is NOTHING like it and I asked God to make his face shine upon me. In prayer later, as I thanked him, these words came into my mind. **"Now you are beginning to know Me, as I AM all around you in all the joyous things I bring to you. The joy you are looking for comes from within you because I AM in you and you are in Me."** I smiled and thanked Him for the message and told him that I wanted to know Him more. I feel that even simple things, like the feel of sunshine on my face, are evidence of God's presence. *Light is sweet, and it pleases the eyes to see the sun. (Ecclesiastes 11:7)*

The little voice, once again, reassured me. I began to look forward even more to praying. I wanted more time alone. What would I hear? So far, the only one I had told was my journal. If this WAS the Lord, He definitely made a habit of communicating directly with me in a non-threatening way. No angel appeared in shining white. No thunder cloud appeared with a booming voice. No giant earthquake or wind storm manifested itself. It was just a small voice in my head that seemed more like my own, sort of like a soft whisper. But, that voice interrupted my thoughts with strong messages that sometimes were repeated over and over.

The Fourth Treatment

I thoroughly enjoyed the time with no chemotherapy treatment, with SOMEONE talking to me in my head. I now dreaded going back for more of the same. It was time for blood work again, which became the weekly routine. I went to the lab, let them stick me in the arm and remove blood for tests a few days before treatment. Then, I went to treatment and received a bigger needle in the other arm. I let the nurse put the IV in the big center vein of my arm so that it burned less. When I arrived for treatment, the nurse told me AGAIN that my white count (now 2.0) and red count dropped even lower, despite the "booster" shots they had given me last time. Did that stop the doctor from giving me a treatment? Did he seem to care that I was going downhill fast? No. This was getting so hard. Is this what God wanted me to do?

The woman in the bed next to me complained about how the Adriamycin she was getting was taking such a bad toll on her. I talked to another patient who had been taking chemo for two years! How did they do it? Obviously, it affects everyone to a different degree. It's definitely not good. The question is, to what degree is it harmful? After only a few treatments, the chemical solution sent worse and worse burning feelings up my arm each time. I watched a woman being brought for chemo in a wheelchair complaining of a bladder and other infections. Egad! Is this what happened after a time? Another woman walked in slowly using a cane and said that the chemotherapy had made her bones brittle and she'd broken a hip. And there I was, receiving another bag of "juice" and another shot to hopefully increase my white cells. Was I simply trading one condition for a different one? Or was I going to add more troubles on top of the one I had? Oh, help me, Lord!

Of course, the nausea returned the following day and my good feeling days were gone for awhile. I slept away the next two days in that abyss while I felt my body getting weaker and weaker. My entire arm still burned where they had inserted the IV. My veins were already affected. Brushing my teeth became something I dreaded because the very act of brushing my teeth, especially in the back, set off the gag reflex. I gagged, brushed some more, gagged some more, brushed, gagged and did the best I could to finish the task.

I researched the different chemotherapy drugs on the internet and didn't like what I saw. The long lasting or permanent side effects listed were more frightening than having cancer—destruction of heart muscle—destruction of the liver—incapacitation of the pancreas. What had I agreed to? *Free me from the net they have set for me, for you are my refuge. Into your hands I commend my spirit, you will redeem me, Lord, faithful God. (Psalm 31:5-6)*

March 5

My hair started falling out today. I hope it doesn't go totally, but I must prepare if it does. I am not afraid. Jesus is with me. I received a message that I am now climbing a mountain. I will reach the top and He will be with me every step of the way. Reminds me of the song that says, "Ain't no mountain high enough to keep me from you." I modified it to say, "Ain't no mountain too high for Jesus and I to climb." STAY with me Lord! *Come, let us climb the Lord's mountain...that he may instruct us in his ways, and we may walk in his paths. (Isaiah 2:3)*

Ok, Lord, I thought. If this IS you talking to me, why are you letting my hair fall out? The nurse told me my hair would not fall out with this medication, and yet, every morning, a good sized clump remained on my pillow. It is rather discouraging to roll over onto your side during the night and feel your face resting on a ball of hair which you know is not the fur of your beloved pet. How could this be happening? I STILL had 14 treatments left! Maybe the hair loss would only occur in the beginning and the rest of my hair would stay intact. There was always hope.

My friend Maggie hated that she had no hair from over one year of enduring chemotherapy treatments. Scarves were now her constant wardrobe accessory, because she could not stand the wigs—too uncomfortable, itchy, and hot. She told me tales of what effect that scarf, and the obvious lack of hair, had on the public. One person in a department store looked at her with great pity and handed her a prayer card. At other places, she would get preferential treatment. Sometimes, people would just stare or go out of their way to avoid contact as if they thought it was contagious. She felt marked with some sign as if people were thinking, "Oh, look! There's another poor soul with cancer, obviously getting chemotherapy." My friend Pat was wearing cute hats and brought me a catalog. I ordered two hats and two scarves from the catalog just in case. I wasn't ready for public sympathy or to feel like an inferior citizen. In retrospect, there was definitely some pride involved on my part.

The Fifth Treatment

This treatment sang the same song, just another verse. Other ladies in the treatment room still looked lifeless. The chemotherapy still burned as it entered my veins with a fire that was now unbelievable. I complained to the nurse about losing my hair and she just said that it happens. My hair got thinner and thinner. I didn't want to wash my hair and see the big clump on the shower floor. Washing my hair seemed to accelerate the process. While reading my Bible, I came across these verses; *Are not five sparrows sold for two copper coins? And yet not one of them is forgotten before God. But, the very hairs on your head are all numbered. Do not fear therefore: you are of more value than many sparrows.(Luke 12:6-7)* I told God it must be pretty easy now to count the remaining hairs on my head. I still made numerous trips to the restroom daily from the aftermath of surgery on my colon. Several books remained in the restroom because it was my second hangout after the couch and the bed.

I fought against letting my brain go wild with bad thoughts. I looked suspiciously at any single woman who brought me food thinking that they were just waiting for me to kick the bucket so they could date my husband. What kind of thoughts were these? This just wasn't the usual "me." Was the "me" that I used to know disappearing? Who or what was I becoming? What kind of statistic in the cancer annals would I be? Would food ever taste good again? Would this cancer drug do some sort of permanent damage? Every time I experienced any pain, I immediately thought the worst. Dark thoughts were abundant. Maggie had talked about planning her funeral, and I chastised her for it, told her to think "life" and not "death." But I almost let my brain begin thinking about that too. Looking back, could this have been the "chemo brain" they spoke of? The next few days contained more queasiness and lots of sleeping.

> March 11
> It is a rainy day today, but I am feeling pretty good and just grateful for everything. When you have a grateful heart, you smile, and when you smile, you can only think good thoughts. You cannot smile and think bad thoughts. It confuses your face. This is part of healing. During prayer today, I told the Lord, "I come to you just as I am and I empty myself. I die to myself and relinquish all to you." Now I know what the apostle Paul meant when he said, *I die daily. (I Corinthians 15:31)* His answer was simple. He said, **"Finally."** I asked Him to fill me with His light and goodness and the light of the Holy Spirit. I know He has begun the process as my body felt a change occurring, almost like the love pangs you get when you are in the beginning of a love relationship. I know I will do great things in His name. Amen.

When I went outside on that rainy day, I actually felt the rain drops hit my scalp. Some drops ran down into my eyes and onto my face. That is how thin my hair was. I also felt any breeze and my head actually got cold. I was discouraged, to say the least. I definitely identify with men who are going bald, but at least their hair doesn't fall out in a matter of a few weeks. A new acquaintance that I met, named Jane, knitted me a scarf and a soft hat to wear to bed at night. The kindness of people again amazed me. The scarves that I purchased from the catalog sat patiently waiting in my dresser drawer, but I refused to use them. I held out. My friends told me to immediately have my head shaved to save myself the agony. I pulled what little hair I had away from my face and looked in the mirror to imagine how my bespectacled face would look with a shaved head. All I saw were glasses and my big Italian nose. The only thing missing to make it one of those funny eyeglasses one bought in the gag store, was a big mustache. I cried my eyes out. I couldn't go let someone shave my head. I just couldn't. I kept repeating to myself, "I have a full head of hair, I have a full head of hair."

> April 5
> I read in a book called God Calling[1] that miracles do not always occur quickly. It took time for Peter to be transformed from someone who denied Jesus three times into a brave person who could go preach. Was that it? Was I learning to be brave? So I asked Jesus how I was being transformed. The answer I received was, **"You are learning patience. You are becoming holier, more like me."** I had never thought of it that way. My spirit is being cured along with my body. Thank you, Lord. I went to the doctor today and he said he is going to lower the concentration of the drugs because of the low blood counts. My white count is now the lowest ever at 1.8. So, Lord, I STILL leave all of this in your hands and am ever so thankful for the great minutes, hours, or days that I do get.

Easter arrived in early April. I wore a hat to church, even though it was a chore to keep it on my head. I never realized that your hair helps keep your hat on. And I purchased all of my Easter bonnets when I had hair. I never even dreamed that they would not stay on my head. I still sported a little hair but it was getting very thin. Even several hat pins did nothing. I could barely sit up in church due to utter exhaustion. Most of the church service, I remained seated with my head on Lloyd's shoulder. All I wanted to do was go to sleep or just lie down. Never had I felt this bad for this long. I was never one to be sick. I felt tremendous pain for those who suffer with long term illnesses. This was so discouraging, yet the Easter message was so encouraging—resurrection, victory over death. I really needed to hear that. *For if we have become united with him in the likeness of his death; certainly we shall also be in the likeness of his resurrection. (Romans 6:5)*

The Sixth Treatment

It was time for another treatment right after Easter. Now that I absolutely knew what to expect, I dreaded it even more. My entire arm ached even before they put the needle in it. I wondered why they bothered with the nausea medicine. And the insurance company was just going to pay another $11,000 plus another $6,000 for a booster shot. Why was I doing this? Because I didn't know what else to do, that's why. Besides, at least my CA-125 was drastically going down, which was encouraging. With this treatment, it was now down to 42—only 21 more to go! So, I took the "lower" dose of the drugs.

The following days repeated the experiences of the weeks before. If they lowered the dose, it must not have been by much. It dawned on me that all they did was experiment. The doctor really didn't know what dosage would work and not kill me. He was winging it. Oh yes, that was comforting. I was now a guinea pig. The tables were sure turned on that one. I used to be a research scientist and now I was the laboratory animal. What was wrong with this? Only my earthly life at stake, that's all.

Betty, my boss at the university, had purchased a book for me entitled *CANCER: 50 ESSENTIAL THINGS TO DO*[2]. The author, Greg Anderson, had interviewed over 15,000 cancer survivors and made a list of what they all had in common. He stated that one must gauge the confidence they have in their medical team. This particularly struck me like a lightning bolt. Anderson also stated that one needs to believe in the treatment program they are experiencing. I had trouble fully believing in the program of chemotherapy from the very beginning. With my brain and body at a low point and only heading lower from more treatments, I was not hopeful. I realized that I had no confidence in the doctor, nor his method of treatment. He had so many women as patients that on autopilot, he simply had a prescribed formula in his head. I needed to change the team or make some sort of change. I knew it in my heart of hearts.

I became weaker, lost more hair, and was just as nauseated. Three days after the treatment, I was unable to stand up without fainting due to the severe anemia and loss of blood cells. My friends tried to tell me to 'suck it up' and tough it out. To me, that wasn't the issue. You 'tough it out' when you believe in it. The couch seemed to have a permanent indentation because of my presence on it day and night. I felt that I could not take much more of this. We only have one sofa and one living room. Lloyd had to sit in a chair.

Please, Lord, I need an answer. I choose to live. *Why do you stand afar off, O Lord? Why do you hide in times of trouble? (Psalm 10:1)*

I continued to pray with great fervor and hoped that the Lord would once again speak to me or that I would hear something. After many times in prayer and prying myself up off the floor, because I would fall asleep while praying, these words came into my head, **"You must stop the chemotherapy. It is going to kill you. I will heal you."** And I doubted and said, "Lord, how do I know this is you talking again and not what I, myself, wish to hear?" All he said was, **"Remember your cat."** (See prologue) A part of me was relieved. No more chemotherapy. But, another part of me was frightened at this revelation. What now? Did I have the nerve to tell this serious and stern looking doctor that I wanted no more part of it? To reject traditional treatment? I've always been a person who avoids conflict or going against the tide. Right now, I needed a dose of confidence and strength.

Mr. Anderson says in his book: "In my opinion, what is happening is that oncologists in the United States are administering chemotherapy to more patients, across a wider spectrum of malignant disease, in the hope that it may show results. The cancer community has tended to extrapolate their narrow successes and consider nearly all cancer patients, especially those with metastatic or recurrent disease, as candidates for chemotherapy. This is the 'why' behind my reservations and this urgent warning to understand clearly what chemotherapy will and will not accomplish."[3] Not only that, but using chemotherapy and radiation on a tumor or tumors is only treating, at best, the SYMPTOM. One or more tumors are only symptoms of something else that has gone wrong in the body. An imbalance is occurring somewhere. Giving only chemotherapy, radiation, and surgery is not addressing, nor trying to heal, the underlying cause.

Heavenly Pearls of Wisdom

Listen. To the encouraging voice inside you. All answers are within and manifested without. (Anything not encouraging is not from a benevolent source.)

Your body does know. It knows what is harmful for it. Discover what you need.

Follow the money and ego trail. Medicine and drugs are big business. Drugs are not always the answer and doctors don't always know.

Do your own research. There are many sources of information. Do not rely on only one. Use the internet and all other resources God places at your disposal.

Chemotherapy is usually NOT the answer. Oncologists are administering more and more chemo with less and less proof of worthwhile results.

3
A Shaft of Light

April 22
I made a decision to stop chemotherapy. I didn't like what I saw on my lab results and read disturbing things about my treatment. Also, my anemia and white counts were getting too low. BUT, tomorrow I have an appointment at the Holistic Clinic and I KNOW that healing has arrived! I am receiving! I asked God to let me know. He has spoken. I just know this was a message from God that all is well. I am cured. I love you, Lord. I believe! *All authority has been given to me in heaven and on earth. (Matthew 28:18).*

I placed a call to the holistic clinic asking if they could accept me yet. Surprisingly, the very day I called, the receptionist said that they were getting ready to call me that day to say that they now had an opening. This clinic takes each patient through a detoxification program. Hallelujah! I was ecstatic. Even though the Lord said he would heal me, I believe that He led me to the clinic to detoxify my body. Wisdom dictates that we take care of our body just as it is wise to take care of our car. *Or do you not know that your body is the temple of the Holy Spirit who is in you, and you are not your own? Glorify God in your body and in your spirit, which are God's. (I Corinthians 6:19-20)*

April 23 was my first appointment. I approached this new endeavor with trepidation and some fear, because I didn't know what to expect. After what I'd been through with chemotherapy, I was apprehensive of what the next type of treatment was going to do to me. The clinic was unassuming enough. It was a set of old homes converted into offices and treatment rooms. I met with the founder and current director, Michele, who very methodically, and yet with compassion, questioned me concerning what I was feeling or what types of systemic problems I was encountering. She did NOT focus on the diagnosis. In fact, she didn't want to dwell on that, which at first I thought odd. There was none of the seriousness and gloom that I had experienced from the doctors. There seemed to me to be an attitude of love, hope and positive expectations. When I later mentioned to my friend Susan how different this atmosphere seemed to be compared to traditional medicine, she explained to me that doctors are trained to have "lowered expectations" and to talk and act with such expectations to the patients. It is purely a protection mechanism in order to protect the medical profession from patients who might say, "But, doctor, you said I would be fine, and now I'm not." I think they have gone a little too far in the other direction, but I do not wish to dwell on that either.

Immediately, the clinic director put me on what I call a unique and individualized "regimen" of changes for health, mind, body, and spirit. Alcohol, sugar, wheat, and dairy (including cheese) were to be eliminated, along with fried foods, red meat and pork, to name a few. What a drastic change that would be in eating! I had started some changes already, but this was drastic! I love Mexican food with all of the cheese as well as Italian food with pasta and more cheese. How could I survive without CHEESE? Michele also created a checklist of all sorts of vitamins and minerals for me to take and the assistants took a hair sample for analysis. They tested my urine and saliva, and sent me for blood chemistry work at a local laboratory. Additionally, the liver detoxification program began.

For I will restore you to health; of your wounds I will heal you, says the Lord. (Jeremiah 30:17)

One of the many problems in using chemotherapy as the sole treatment, and any pill or set of pills that are prescribed, is that they merely treat symptoms of disease. Many doctors prescribe chemotherapy for a person and then the person makes no other changes. They eat the same foods as before and are probably lacking in the same minerals and vitamins, if not more, after the prescribed chemical treatment begins. The issue of side effects arises which causes more prescriptions to be added. People continue with the same habits, content with their handful of pills and fill their minds, bodies, and souls with the same previous thoughts. People need change from the inside out.

Each Monday evening, the clinic founder, Michele Longo O'Donnell, author of the book mentioned in this paragraph, speaks to all patients and any other interested people. It is definitely not a "woe is me" type of encounter. Each week contains a message of wholeness and goodness and the mercy of the Lord. She focuses on those things and not on a "sickness." Most of the patients have read her book, *Of Monkeys and Dragons: freedom from the Tyranny of Disease*[1]. We were taught to give no power to the things of this world which attempt to come up against us and declare themselves to be a power. There is only ONE power and that is God. *But if the Spirit of Him who raised Jesus from the dead dwells in you, He who raised Christ from the dead will also give life to your mortal bodies through His Spirit who dwells within you. (Romans 8:11).* I am still attending these meetings to this day.

We were encouraged by the clinic and Michele to read our Bible, listen to praise and worship music, and to guard our minds and thoughts. I quit reading the paper, did not read the obituaries, only watched the weather on the news and did not watch any horror movies or read horror books. In fact, I stopped the paper delivery completely. After all, of what benefit would they be? I was already fearful and those things would only make it worse. When I did rent a movie, it was a comedy.

All of a sudden one realizes how much time has been wasted watching television, reading junk magazines, clamoring over information on politicians and celebrities, playing video games, reading "trash" novels, and many other activities that occupy our minds and to what avail? *It is all vanity and a chase in the wind. (Ecclesiastes 2:17)* When I added up the time spent in totally unfruitful ways, it was shocking. Yet, the populace is surrounded and inundated with it all. And whatever is taken in, be it good or horrific, enters the subconscious, and works continuously in the mind, even while a person sleeps. That is one of the reasons that dreams incorporate events from your recent day or days.

In comparison, how much time is spent in silence, talking with the Lord, praying, reading words of wisdom, enjoying nature, or just entertaining thankful and grateful thoughts? The Bible contains words and phrases that jumped out of the page and spoke directly to me. I wrote many of them down in my journal or a notebook and focused on them. I wrote some of them on a piece of paper and pinned it to the bathroom wall. A shaft of light was beginning to pierce the darkness. Thank you, Lord, for your Word. One of the recognized Catholic saints, St. Teresa of Avila, in her book entitled, *The Interior Castle,*[2] states that our souls are like a crystal castle with a drawbridge, and God at the center. When those undesirable influences or thoughts try to act upon you, close the drawbridge quickly! Go into the castle and run to the center. Be with God.

April 29
Monday was my first appointment at the Holistic clinic—Hooray! Michele O'Donnell is the director, and she set me up with an individual plan for eating, taking herbs, drinking fresh carrot, celery, apple juice, and more. I've gone to the clinic every day. Priscilla helped me with the first treatment since I was so afraid. She is awesome. Thank you, Lord, that

she was the first technician I saw there. The liver and body must be cleansed of yeast, parasites, metals and other toxins. I firmly believe the Lord sent me here as an answer to my prayer and my desire to choose life and live deliberately. My hope is in the Lord. His words came to me, **"It is I, I your Lord, who has healed you."** Thank you, Jesus. The juicing and other items take up much of my day, but I read that miracles done by Jesus, in many cases, required some effort on the part of the one being healed. The blind man had to go wash the mud from his eyes. So, I'm doing my part as the miracle of healing occurs.

Jesus said, **"It is time for your resurrection."** Do you know what that means? It means that it is time for the suffering to be OVER! Hallelujah! Resurrection to health, my body being whole, perfect, strong, powerful, in harmony, happy, and loving! It HAS arrived.

Rising Up

Within a week, I was beginning to feel much better physically and mentally. The fogginess and confusion began to dissipate. My mind and body responded in a great way to everything. My body seemed to be craving natural substances. After purchasing a good heavy duty juicer, I was pleased to discover that I actually liked freshly squeezed carrot, celery, apple, and spinach juice mixed together! Looking back in my journal, it was so arrogant of me to think that I couldn't "get into that." Well, I'm definitely "into it" with both feet! The exact proportions that I use to this day are: 16 ounces of fresh carrot juice (about 9 good-sized carrots), 2 ounces of celery juice (two stalks), 1-2 ounces of spinach (a large handful) or parsley juice, and one entire apple—all organic and washed. A heavy duty juicer must be purchased. I tried the cheap one and it gave out after only 2 or 3 juicings. (I purchased a Breville™.) I pour the remains out onto the yard in back. The pulp is returned to nature and not to a landfill. There are people "on the program," as it is called, who take their juicer to work and do their juicing there. I used to think those fresh juices were only for the "hippie" types.

Getting fresh enzymes to individual body cells was an amazing thought to me. My body no longer received a dose of poison, but life-giving nutrition. It was rewarding to work in conjunction with my body systems instead of against them. Although I once had been a chemistry teacher, I didn't fully realize how important enzymes were to the functioning of the body and in keeping foreign invaders under control. Where are those enzymes? Only in fresh fruits and vegetables. Most people who go grocery shopping don't even have one fresh fruit or vegetable in their cart at checkout. (It's been a hobby of mine to look at other people's carts now that I heard that.) I am shocked to see some people come to the checkout with nothing but crates of sodas, beer, processed foods, and snacks. Previously, I had occasionally eaten fresh fruits and sometimes lettuce and tomato. But, most of the time, I ingested TV dinners because I worked late. Or I turned to frozen pizzas, fast food, and once in a while I actually cooked a meal. Lloyd worked nights and both of my daughters were on their own. There was not much incentive to cook when I was tired after a day of work.

Eating and drinking in a way that includes mostly processed and fast food, one generation becomes deficient in the necessary enzymes. In their advancing years, people get cancer, arthritis, diabetes, and many other illnesses. They unknowingly pass any deficiency on to their children and the children eat like the parents, becoming even more deficient (second generation) in minerals and enzymes, getting those diseases in mid-years. These children grow up and have children who are now born with more extreme enzyme deficiencies (third generation) and with severe health problems. They may even crave unusual foods such as pickles or non-food items such as chalk or talcum powder. Even craving chocolate may be indicative of a deficiency. Cancer and many other diseases were never known among children to the degree they are presently. Cancer is the number one killer of children today. Now, babies are born with problems or develop them shortly thereafter. We must watch what we take into our body. We are not just feeding our own bodies but the generations to come after us.

Fears to Overcome

It was wonderful to start feeling good again and see no more hair falling out. But, could it be true? Was this really the right choice? Was everything just being postponed? These were the fears that began to snake around my mind like the serpent speaking to Adam and Eve, attempting to crush the successes like a boa constrictor. I excitedly told someone about my clinic detoxification treatment and she was absolutely not in favor of it, even said it was dangerous. How was it more dangerous than chemotherapy? But, my doubt grew and I prayed.

> May 3
> I talked with someone who doesn't believe in holistic treatment such as this. So, I prayed and the message I heard very clearly was this: **"Continue on; My hand is over all."** Thank you Lord, as difficult as it is, I will trust you. *When I am afraid, I will put my trust in you. In God, whose word I praise, in God I have put my trust; I shall not be afraid. What can mere man do to me? (Psalm 56:3-4)*

Part of my quest became to read as much as possible about cancer, disease, nutrition, health, and spirituality. I became a hungry-for-knowledge reading fool. I read day and night, whenever I wasn't working. I stumbled upon the advice of Dr. Lorraine Day[3] on the internet and adopted her 10 habits for returning to health. I have included most of them at the end of this and upcoming chapters. I continued taking short 10-15 minutes walks outdoors after my surgery and the weather was actually quite nice. The air felt refreshing and I took deep breaths, soaking up the life-renewing air and sunlight. The clinic had recommended getting a personal-sized trampoline. Apparently, jumping on a trampoline for at least two minutes greatly helps the lymphatic system move things along. This helps clear the body of foreign matter that has been attacked and broken down. I definitely planned to buy one.

Every source I found stressed drinking water to help with all body functions and to remove toxins from the body. The recommendation was 64 ounces. The clinic regulated this for me. At first, I measured it out exactly as instructed. Then, it became more instinctual and my body gave me signs when it did not get enough water for the day.

May 17

I went to the oncologist today and excitedly told him about my holistic program. He pretty much condemned the whole thing. I left there feeling devastated spiritually and mentally. I forgave him for being so discouraging, but I cannot go back to him or that depressing place where they give the chemotherapy. I really prayed a lot and Jesus has said so much to me that I can't remember it all to write it down. But he did say, **"Soon, I will give you an outward sign of your healing."** Lord I hold on to that and wait patiently. And forgive me for the times my faith waivers. I get weak in my humanness.

The devil tries to sow doubt and despair, but I REJECT that and go to the light of the Lord. Tomorrow, I am going to a different doctor recommended by my boss, Betty. I'd really like to get another opinion or find a doctor with an open mind. I pray for support. The Holistic Health Care people are so positive and supportive and believe in the Lord and his power.

I must practice seeing myself as whole, perfect, healthy, happy, and holy! I am grateful to you, O Lord! Continue to help me and do not abandon me.

I bought a mini trampoline and the first time I used it, I wet my pants! I'm going to have to get stronger bladder muscles!

❧Shaft of Light Narrows❧

I showed up for my scheduled doctor check up, just like the nurse had advised me to do a few weeks prior. I entered feeling physically good and joyful. I wanted to share with the doctor what I had "discovered".

"Good afternoon, Diana. How are you feeling?" asked the doctor as he examined me inside and out.

"Doctor, I feel really GREAT!' I said enthusiastically.

"Do you really?" he asked with his eyebrows raised as if he didn't believe me.

"I certainly do!" I replied joyously. "I started a program at the holistic clinic and it is wonderful!"

"Is that so? Well, I don't know anything about this clinic and I've seen lots of ladies die trying the natural route," he stated sarcastically. All of a sudden, while examining me, he stopped abruptly and stated, "Your lymph glands are extremely swollen in the groin area here. They are probably full of cancer."

"No, the clinic told me they might swell up from the detoxification process. They'll be fine," I said with some confidence.

"They will not be fine. They are full of cancer and we need to take you to surgery immediately so that I can remove them." He stated this emphatically and with a sense of urgency.

"I'm not letting you take out my lymph nodes. I know what happens. My legs will permanently swell up like elephant legs because the lymph pools in them. No way. No surgery. They will be fine."

"You are making a mistake. They are full of cancer," he argued with great conviction. "And besides that, what is this program all about?" He was definitely in the non-believing mode after viewing and feeling my almond sized lymph nodes.

"It's a great program, doctor, one that works to heal the immune system and detoxify the liver," I said as I tried to begin explaining.

"Why did you decide to do that? You need to finish the chemotherapy." This was said with emphasis like it was a certainty.

"Well, you will probably think this is strange, but I received a message in prayer to stop the chemotherapy or it would kill me."

He snorted and said, "God doesn't talk to people. He hasn't done that since the time of Abraham and Moses. Besides that, I talk to God all of the time and He never talks to ME."

My heart was sinking rapidly as I tried once more to explain. "But, I know I received this in prayer."

"And I've seen lots of women die praying, too," came the matter-of-fact reply. "I've been dong this for 30 years and I've seen it all."

I became physically ill to my stomach. What could I say next? I gave it one more try. "But, doctor, I feel so good! I have energy and my hair isn't falling out like before."

"Feeling good means nothing," came the startling reply. Then he picked up his pen and began to write. "I'm writing your prescription for the next chemotherapy session next week."

"Doctor, I'm NOT taking any more chemotherapy! I'm going to try something else." My heart was pounding wildly as I confronted him.

"If it were me, *I'd* take the chemo."

"You would?" I found that difficult to believe considering the suffering he must surely witness by giving it to his patients.

"Yes, I would."

"It's just not for me. I know there has got to be a better way."

His pen stopped writing and he looked at me with sadness and resignation. "I'd still like to be your doctor, no matter what you decide."

What a dichotomy that seemed to be. I stood up and started walking out. "Ok, I'll think about it," I said dejectedly—when pigs fly, I thought to myself. I never returned. He probably thinks

I'm dead. I wonder what that did to the chemo statistics. If the chemotherapy kills the cancer cells and the patient dies, the treatment is still considered successful. I'm probably labeled as "status unknown—dropped out of study." He did a fantastic job on my surgery and for that I give him credit and thanks. I'm glad I never let him take out my lymph glands. They are back down to normal size now. I continue to pray for him and only wish him well. Everyone arrives at the truth on different time schedules. I wasn't living his time schedule, but my own.

Adriana Trigiani, one of my favorite Italian fiction writers, said it best in the 3rd book of her trilogy, *Milk Glass Moon*. She stated about a woman she met, "...I will never see her again. We met when we had to, and our business is done." [4]

Though our business was, to me, finished, I cannot begin to tell you how the words of the doctor set me back. *Give not that which is holy unto the dogs, neither cast ye your pearls before swine, lest they trample them under their feet, and turn again and rend you. (Matthew 6:7)* I had thrown my pearls before swine. My spirits rapidly sank to a new low. This was a respected physician and surgeon. As a society, we are taught to revere them. How could he be saying this? I guess I can't blame him for what he has embraced, but I didn't understand his unwillingness to even listen to anything alternative.

The sleepless nights returned. Fear began to overtake my mind. Was the doctor correct? Was I going to die? Was this all a cruel joke on me? Was this "test of faith" business just another cliché? Had I failed it if it was a test? My heart cried out to the Lord.

Additionally, during that time, my brother-in-law, Myron, was ailing from all of the treatments he had received. The radiation had so badly burned his esophagus that it was extremely irritated and raw, closing off as a food passage. With no way to get nutrition, the VA hospital inserted a stomach tube. Also, my friend Maggie, who had now been on chemotherapy for more than 8 months, experienced numbness in her feet and hands, could not use the computer anymore, and could barely walk, all of these horrible side effects from the treatment. My friend Pam, who received the blood transfusions, was now receiving radiation treatments and still feeling very tired and worn out, in addition to being frightened at the breast surgery to come. What was happening? Destruction was all around me. My mind reeled with the senselessness of it all. *A thousand shall fall at thy side, and ten thousand at thy right hand, but it shall not come nigh thee. (Psalm 91:7)*

Going to the clinic several times a week actually helped me through all of this. Melissa, the assistant director, encouraged me and told me that no one knew when someone's body was going to die except God. She helped me realize that I did not have to accept what the doctor had said even though his words repeated over and over in my head, like a damaged CD that plays the same track repeatedly until you switch to another track. Switching to another track was very difficult when fear was winding its whispery tendrils around me. She said not to internalize those words and ideas but to internalize that I was a beautiful and perfect creature created in the image and likeness of God. After much praying, filling my head with positive things, and pushing all of the negativity away from me, I began to have renewed hope.

> May 20
> I had a beautiful Mother's Day! I love being with family—just love it. Jesus, thank you for family and people who love us. Thank you for calmness and happiness in families when it is there, for however long.

Fortunately, my husband, daughters, and parents supported my decision to follow a holistic approach. After one has prayed and received an answer or intuition from the Lord about the best path to health, we must avoid the toxic relatives and friends who do not support the decision. I witnessed at least two patients at the clinic whose own spouses did not support them in the program. Imagine coming home every day and your spouse or someone else close to you tells you that you've made a bad choice, that you are not looking good, that you might as well give up. How long could you withstand that?

This is the time to be firm and confident in the decision, even though it might be difficult. If our spouses, children, or parents truly love us, then we must impress upon them the importance of their support in this life or death matter, or at least to remain quiet. Get back in the castle. *Seek the Lord and his strength, seek his presence continually! (I Chronicles 16:11)*

> May 21
> Went to a new doctor today who explained why a doctor can't violate medical codes by endorsing any type of holistic treatment. But, he did give me a prayer sheet. He said that he has seen DRAMATIC improvement with dramatic changes in diet! That was encouraging because I've definitely made a drastic change there. He was such a nice man. I wish many blessings upon him. He gave me several helpful things.
>
> While jumping on my trampoline, I heard these words, **"Spend time with me. I am your sanctuary."** I want to spend even more time conversing with You, Lord! I want to enter the castle and experience you there. Thank you, thank you for miracles!

Yes, I saw a different doctor that I'd heard was very compassionate, understanding, and willing to consider alternatives. People always tell you to get a second opinion, so I tried my best to do just that. This man, Doctor W, told me that the medical profession, the FDA (Food and Drug Administration), and the drug companies have a VERY tight hold on the individual doctors. If they so much as even consider publicly endorsing any type of holistic, herbal, or alternative program, they are in danger of losing their license. So, he did not officially endorse the program I was following, yet he informed me, his very own daughter was in such a program at an institute in Austin, Texas. Aha! Another small shaft of light! He secretly believed! I wondered how many other doctors there are who know of natural alternatives and yet, are too afraid to embrace them publicly for fear of being "lynched" by their colleagues or being subverted by the drug companies. And, they do not learn any of this in medical school. What has happened to our society? Why do we accept this? Why don't we rise up and complain?

He agreed to order a CA-125 and any other blood tests that I wanted. Then he said something strange but interesting. "Wait here, I think I have something for you." Was it a medication or what? He returned with three sheets of paper, which he handed to me. The first contained the name and web site of the holistic institute in Austin. The second sheet contained the name of a book, *Entering the Castle: An Inner Path to God and your Soul*, by Caroline Myss.[5] It is based on the book by St. Theresa I mentioned earlier but actually takes you through specific spiritual exercises. And the third sheet contained three prayers for healing. Those touched my heart. What a difference compared to the last doctor. He was not an oncologist.

"Thank you for these, doctor. I really appreciate the information," I said, as I jumped off of the exam table and prepared to leave his office.

As he was walking out of the room, he turned and said to me, "You need to go there." He pointed to the pages I now held in my hand.

"Go where? To the holistic institute in Austin?" I asked.

"No, THERE!" he stated emphatically as he pointed to the title of the book.

"Into the castle?" I asked, bewildered.

"Yes," he replied as he left.

"Ok, I'll check it out. Thanks again. I know that you did what you felt you were able to for me."

"You're welcome."

I felt that a new adventure into my relationship with God awaited me. After I paid my bill, I left somewhat saddened that this doctor couldn't really help me as much as I wanted, due to the restrictions placed on him by his own peers. This is a sad state that costs human lives and health. I truly had to rely on the Lord who was indeed directing my path. *Commit your way to the Lord; trust in him, and he will act. (Psalm 37:5)* I ran to the nearest bookstore and purchased Carolyn Myss's book he'd recommended. I performed the spiritual and meditational exercises in her book and it was one of the best things I've ever done in my life.

Later in the week, one of my real estate clients from England, Olwen, asked me to go shopping with her to the local mall and I gladly accepted. Shopping! It used to be one of my favorite past times when I actually had money to spend! All the striking colors of clothing and other items on display seemed to soothe the spirit. I had missed the experience....even though now I looked, but didn't feel as much desire to buy. My priorities had changed and so had my body shape. I still had a tender scar running the length of my torso, hardly had any hair on my head, and felt self conscious trying on any clothes. But, it was glorious to get out and see all of the pretty things. Olwen is so much fun and most encouraging. She is a cancer survivor herself.

To my amazement, while we were aimlessly wondering through an electronics and gadgetry store, I ran into a friend of mine that I once worked with. She moved to Arizona a few years ago and I had not seen her since. We greeted one another, hugged and embraced. She seemed friendly, but not quite her old vivacious self for some reason. She told me that she and her husband had returned to the city for a short visit and were trolling the mall while they waited to go to the airport and catch a plane home. So, I told her what had happened to me with the diagnosis I'd been given, expecting, I think, some sort of surprise and sympathy. Her reaction totally changed my life.

She said, "I've been there and come back from that." But, she still had sadness in her eyes. I expressed my sympathy and surprise and marveled at how well she looked. I asked how her only child and 24 year-old namesake daughter was doing, who they affectionately called "junior." Immediately, a cloud came over her face and with tears that welled up in her eyes, she told me, "My daughter was killed in an auto accident 2 years ago." Stunned, I stammered around and did not know what to say except that I was sorry. She had faced cancer AND the death of her only child. Life was so cruel to people, it seemed. I held her and we both cried. This was definitely like being in someone else's bad dream.

I will always remember her parting words to me. She said, "Diana, whatever you do, *never* own this diagnosis. Do not call it 'my cancer'. It is not of you and has no part of you. Disown it immediately." I made a decision to embrace that advice. My thanks to her, my friend, for she had reached out and brought light to me, even after she had descended into her own time of darkness.

May 23
This is what I heard today. **"You will be one of my many miracles. Then, you can tell others, just like the man who was blind did."** I believe. I am receiving the healing of the Holy Spirit. I surrender to Jesus first and then the Holy Spirit.

I went to a dinner this evening and met Melinda, a woman who went into a coma for 5 weeks for no apparent reason. During that time, she had many conversations with the Lord and then miraculously, came out of the coma after the hospital and her family had given her up for lost. Thank you, Lord, for your encouragement and the stories of hope. You are awesome.

Every time I went anywhere, I met people who had their own story to tell, but this one let me know that I was not crazy, that God did indeed talk to people......even me. I had so much to learn and felt that so many years of my life had unconsciously slipped away. *Make me to know your ways, O Lord; teach me your paths. (Psalm 25:4)*

Heavenly Pearls of Wisdom

Guard your mind. Let only good thoughts nest there.

Guard your body. It does matter what you do or don't give it.

Get outside in the sunshine and fresh air. They have healing properties. It's not just a myth.

Drink water. At least 56 to 64 ounces. No tea or soda.

Buy a good juicer and juice fresh vegetables. Your body will thank you many times over.

Get some form of MILD exercise. Avoid vigorous exercise as it stresses the body too much.

Do NOT own a diagnosis. Do not call it my this or my that. Give it no power at all. It is not of you.

Keep a circle of support. Talk to a small group of encouraging people and close the circle tight. Don't listen to detractors.

4
Appearance of Grace

May 24
Today this message was given to me, **"You will be a light as I am the light of the world and you are a branch of that light. Do not despair—have hope and trust in me. You are my gift. Live for me. Do my will—be that light in continual health."**

Answering Religious Clichés

One of the difficult things when dealing with something serious was the clichés that people said to me without really thinking about them. The one that used to bother me was, "If it is God's will, you will be healed." Why would it NOT be God's will? I read my Bible every day. Nowhere in those pages did I read that Christ said no to anyone who asked to be healed. He even approached them and asked if they wanted to be healed. I never read anything like this, "No, I don't think it's my Father's will nor mine for you to be healed today!" I read several sources that said not to pray to the Lord just to whine about being healed, but to humbly CLAIM a healthy body, mind, and spirit as our rightful inheritance. Once we are in tune with God, His will and our will are one and the **same**. There is no conflict in that because the heart, soul, and mind are in unison with the mind of God.

May 25

I got the results of my CA-125 today. It was up a little to 22 from the last one of 16 but I was expecting that. I refuse to focus on a number! I know I am in God's hands and I believe that this holistic program works! But, I also believe in the truth: God made us in His image and likeness, whole and perfect. He wants us that way. It is his will for us. Jesus, I claim total healing and health! I wait for the outward sign. It will come!

May 28

"You are free. Cling to the truth, Diana. Cling to the truth of my power, my power over ALL forces, even those of which man has no knowledge. When you surrender to me, I am in charge. What you have asked is my will for you."

May 29

Jesus, when the soldiers came to arrest you in the garden of Gethsemane, an apostle cut off the ear of a soldier, and you immediately healed him. So, you even healed people who meant to do you harm. I know you have healed me, because, even though I have sinned against you in the past, your love and mercy endure toward ALL. I await the outward sign. **"Be still and know that I am here. Quiet your mind. Breathe in my Holy Spirit, breathe out what is not of Me. Breathe in my Holy Spirit, breathe out all darkness. Breathe in my Holy Spirit, breath out all that is past. Breathe in my Holy Spirit, breathe out all doubts. Breathe in my Holy Spirit, breathe out my Holy Spirit upon others. My mind is joined with yours. Take peace and harmony with you. It is in you. It is not dependent upon external forces."** Thank you, Lord, for all. My heart is grateful. Oh, Lord, I seek to know you and be in touch with my soul—to enter into my castle— but I don't know how. **"I will help you. Continue to be grateful, for that opens the door. Abide in me. Allow my grace to flow through you."** *...for it is time to seek the Lord. (Hosea 10:12)*

I reiterate the point here that Jesus healed one who had come to arrest him. Why would he not want to see me and others healed too? He even asked for mercy upon those who put him to death. But Jesus was saying, *Father forgive them; for they do not know what they are doing. (Luke 23:34)*

And I particularly took comfort when I came across this passage, *Or who among you would hand his son a stone when he asks for a loaf of bread, or a snake when has asks for a fish? If you, then, who are wicked, know how to give good gifts to your children, how much more will your father in heaven give good things to those who ask him! (Matthew 7:9-11)* I realized that God WANTS to grant us health and all good things.

Another cliché I heard often was, "If God led you to it, He will lead you through it." God did NOT lead me to this! God is only goodness and mercy. He does not lead us to these things. Many things we do or what we are surrounded by lead us to these situations. As I read more of His words, I became even more convinced of this in my heart. It is the darkness of man's thinking that has brought us here, along with the invention of items that intentionally or unintentionally destroy man. Once Adam and Eve ate the forbidden fruit, thus began the appearance of evil and dark thinking. *But from the tree of the knowledge of good and evil you shall not eat, for in the day you eat from it you shall surely die. (Genesis 2:17)*

And the third and final cliché I do not listen to is, "Let go and let God." Earlier, I said that the first thing to do is pray. The second is to listen for God's answer and it WILL come. Joel Goldsmith, in his book entitled *The Master Speaks,* states, "This is not an attitude of 'let God do it', since that would involve a sense of separation from God....it is not with resigned acceptance that 'whatever happens God did it'; or 'I will take whatever God sends me.' Such an attitude is duality."[1] To me, and after listening to Michele's words, we are one with God. He works through us and WITH us. We make space for the Lord to do his work in and through us. That doesn't mean that we do nothing at all or think nothing, but once we have made the space, we wait for God's direction to come in and through us. It might come through something that is read, a phone call, something seen or heard, an idea that just seems to "pop" into your head, the direct voice in your head, a gut feeling, something a person says to you, or in any number of various ways. You will just know that it is what you are supposed to be aware of and do.

Healing Through Gratefulness

Giving thanks and expressing gratefulness to the Lord every day was also good for my spirit. Thank him for the body systems that ARE working, rather than concentrating on those that aren't working at one hundred percent capacity. I start each day, from the minutes of awakening, thanking God for something. I began with simple things such as being thankful for food, a good night's sleep, clothing, a home, people who love me, being able to talk and sing, and so on. I focus on the positive and give thanks. If a friend calls me, I give thanks. If the garbage disposal works, give thanks. If the car is working, thank Him. If fears leave, give thanks. One could actually make a pretty extensive list of things for which to be thankful. It's not a one time event that happens in November. It is CONSTANT. How could God not be moved to heal a grateful heart? *Be anxious for nothing, but in everything by prayer and supplication, with* ***thanksgiving****, let your requests be made known to God. (Philippians 4:6)* Be thankful always.

June 4

"Continue to get to know me. Read my word and reflect. It will have meaning for you. You are asking for guidance. It will come when you are ready. I grant you my grace and

it will continue to change you. I provide you with what you need. At times, you do not know what you need but I provide—just as a young child does not know that he needs vitamins and the parents provide them."

Focus On and Bless Others

A healthy spirit is led to think about other people, pray for them, send them healing, and send them grace. Imagine yourself heaping grace and God's love upon others. When people asked me what they could do for me during my time of crisis, I told them to send me a get well card in the regular mail. This accomplished four things. First, I had to walk to the mailbox and retrieve the mail so I got at least 2 blocks worth of exercise, sunshine, and fresh air. Second, the cards made me feel really good and I knew that someone thought of me long enough to buy the card, write the card, and send the card. Third, I went through those cards one by one several times in the months ahead and each time I read the name of the person(s) who signed the card, I felt the presence of grace and the love of the Lord for them. I wished many blessings upon them. Fourth, it forced me to take the focus off of myself and my fears, and focus on someone else. Keep in mind that whatever health crisis you face, others around you are also being affected in many ways. Bless them all.

Nutrition and Air

As mentioned earlier, a DRASTIC change in diet started my treatment program. It was very difficult, especially if Lloyd and I wanted to dine out. Another drastic change that I had to make was to eliminate as much wheat from my diet as possible. How can this be, you ask yourself? Everything we read says to eat whole wheat bread, whole wheat pasta, and all sorts of wheat products. There is only one problem with that advice. The world is not what it once was, including the produce and grains. As the years have advanced, growers and processors have made subtle changes. One such change was to genetically breed a thicker hybrid wheat grain. This produced more wheat gluten, which is a thick sticky substance. Therefore, it took less wheat to make breads because the increased gluten gave it more substance and allowed it to rise better. But, wheat gluten, being the sticky substance that it is, sticks to our insides, and is not digested well. People began to develop inflammations or allergies to this new gluten, even though many are still not yet aware that gluten is causing their allergy symptoms. If a body is trying to rebuild itself, along with re-arming its immune system, or ridding itself of a disease like cancer, it is unable to do so if the immune system is reacting to an allergen, such as gluten. So, what is the solution? The answer is to either avoid wheat products altogether or to try spelt.

What is spelt? It is simply a type of wheat grain the way that it used to be as far back as ancient times. I find spelt bread, rolls, pasta, and a number of spelt products at the local health food store. One can even bake with spelt flour. It is more easily digested, has higher protein, and may not produce the allergies that our current wheat products do. Personally, I like the taste of spelt because it tastes similar to whole wheat. Of course, if you are Italian like me, we may not be able to find spelt ravioli, manicotti, and ziti. If you have Celiac disease, you are cautioned against using spelt also. But, for the rest of us, switching to spelt can help greatly. Millet is another product that one can substitute. *Take wheat and barley, beans and lentils,* ***millet*** *and* ***spelt;*** *put them in a storage jar and use them to make bread for yourself. (Ezekiel 4:9)*

During surgery recovery and continuing on into other treatments, I engaged in breathing exercises of Dr. Andrew Weil,[2] given to me on CD from Angela. I loved how my children helped me. Even if one can't exercise, deep breathing exercises are a possibility. The body loves the intake of air and oxygen. It assists with healing of tissues and interestingly enough, is loathed by cancer cells. They have mutated and adapted to an anaerobic (without oxygen) environment. Cancer cells actually use sugar for their energy supply instead of oxygen like other normal cells do. The theory is that this allows them to thrive in an acid environment in a body that is also not getting enough oxygen to the tissues.

A simple breathing exercise that I did several times a day was to sit or lie down in a relaxed position. Inhale deeply while counting slowly to four. Hold the breath while slowly counting to seven. Then, slowly let the breath out to the count of eight, while holding the tongue to the roof of the mouth just behind the front top teeth. Do this exercise just four times each session and no more. It is also calming and relaxing for the body. *Then the Lord God formed man of the dust from the ground, and breathed into his nostrils the breath of life, and man became a living being. (Genesis 2:7)*

God gives you information so that you can act when you are supposed to. Do what you can as you are led by the Lord. He WILL guide you IF you ask. So many times, he revealed to me, people do not ask for guidance or mercy. ASK!!! He wants us to.

A Different Test of Faith

June 5
I received word today through Lloyd that Matthew Kuglic's parents called and said that he was killed by an explosive device in Kirkuk, Iraq. My heart is heavy, I've cried all day, and I grieve the loss. I know I should not ask why, but why? Oh, God, be with his family—give them comfort. I love you, Matthew, like a son. I pray for Les and Donna and Emily. No family should have to bear this.

I was inconsolable. Here was a young man, my client and friend, mature, Christian, very dedicated to the service of his country, who visited me in the hospital.....and he was gone. We had previously met his parents when they visited him at the air force base here. How could this be? Was it real? What sort of darkness is in the world and in the hearts of men to blow up their fellow humans who are only trying to help them? The military gave him a most honorable tribute and acknowledged his family in the stands on the field of the air base. Why him, Lord? Only 24 years old. You gave me a second (or maybe third or fourth) chance. Why didn't he get a second chance? I cried more than I could remember crying in a long time. His mom and dad had sent me pictures of him dancing with the Iraqi children and families. When asked why he was so willing to go to a foreign country to fight a devious and elusive enemy, he had replied, "I do it for them, the children."

How could I concentrate on healing and the Lord? Where were all my grandiose thoughts about blessing people now? No wonder nations are at war for years over the atrocities that they do to each other. Oh, my God...help me. My faith was shattered that day. Nothing made sense in this world. *All was well with me, but he shattered me; he seized me by the neck and crushed me. (Job 16:12)*

> June 8
> Matthew, pray for us all still here. The news of Matthew is no easier today. Matthew, no good-byes—only an "I'll see you later." I still remember our last e-mail communication. He had asked me what forgiveness entailed. I had prayed, asked for inspiration from the Holy Spirit, and sent him a reply. He graciously thanked me and that was the last I heard from him. My spirit cries out to you, God.

Slowly, I came out from under this cloud, but I will always feel a special fondness for Matthew and his family. They say time heals all, but I believe that for a tragedy of this magnitude it merely dulls the pain a little. When Matthew's box of possessions arrived from overseas, his parents told me there was a gift for me, a box of prayer beads. I cried again. Several months later, when his military group finished a mission, his parents told me that he had wanted Lloyd and me to have the American flag from that mission. When they flew down for another memorial service and presented that flag to us, my heart cried with a mixture of joy and agony. Why am I telling this? To share with you that no journey to healing is ever without obstacles. To show that sadness still can occur in our lives. How will Matthew's family ever heal? During those times, relying on the Lord brings more comfort than turning our backs on Him. God did not do this; the evil in men's hearts did this. *Be merciful to me, O Lord, for I am in distress; my eyes grow weak with sorrow, my soul and my body with grief. (Psalm 31:9)* May his sacrifice never be forgotten and may he be dancing with Jesus and the children in heaven.

> June 28
> I pray for grace, Jesus-grace to have faith, grace to heal, grace to help others, divine grace.

I felt strong and well enough to take a yoga class at the gym. Can you believe it, after only three months on the holistic program? The yoga music was soothing and healing. Apparently, some of the sound waves have a profound effect on the body in terms of healing. My body hurt the next day at first. I pulled a few groin muscles and the fear returned that something was wrong with me. Why did I allow my mind to go crazy with those kinds of thoughts? Because I still had trouble believing that God wanted me healed? People may think they don't deserve all good things, or do not trust either the decision they made, or the Lord to help them, or both.

My favorite part of yoga is at the end, after you've worked muscles that you forgot you had, stretched some very tight muscles, and been twisted up into all sorts of contorted positions, you get to lie flat on your back and just rest. At first I didn't like the fact that they called it the "corpse pose." I wished they would rename it. I was trying to focus on living, not dying. In any case, I certainly enjoyed it. I felt like the music was penetrating my whole body and filling it with white healing light. I would highly recommend some form of this if you can handle it—both for men and women. The movements are slow and the breathing deep, which is quite a contrast to our shallow-breathing fast-paced world. To this day, I attend yoga or similar types of classes at the local gym.

Learning to Believe

July 3

"You are thinking right. You are acting right. It shall come. What you wish for is yours—continue to claim. Continue on the path I set before you. My hand is over all. Act in faith. Love in faith. Be glad. My light is in every cell of your body. Feel my light." I prayed and asked the Lord what I should read in the Bible. He said to read Psalm 13. I was surprised at what it said and how well it applied to me. *Look upon me, answer me, Lord, my God. I trust in your faithfulness, grant my heart joy in your help, that I may sing of the Lord. How good our God has been to me! (Psalm 13:1,6)*

When people would ask me how I was doing, of course, I answered that I was doing great. They would say that I looked fabulous, even though I had a distinct orange color from the liver detoxification and the fresh carrot juice I drank twice a day. Then, they would marvel at the work and sacrifice it takes to be on a holistic program and say things like, "I don't know if I could ever do all of that," or "That's just too much to do and too many foods to give up!" But, what I never told them was that giving up alcohol, chocolate, certain foods, doing juicing, and so on was the EASY part. The hardest part was having consistent, constant FAITH and TRUST that all would be well. I wavered. I would be strong for a few days and afraid for the next several days. I would wake up in the middle of the night and fear would overtake me. How was this fear to be overcome? I prayed, I sang hymns, and I read the Bible. I talked to other people attending the clinic who seemed pretty confident. And I prayed some more. I prayed for the strength to BELIEVE. *...as you have believed, let it be done for you. (Matthew 8:13).* I believe God took away the fear and the

Holy Spirit did the praying for me. *In the same way, the Spirit helps us in our weaknesses. We do not know what we ought to pray for, but the Spirit himself intercedes for us with groans that words cannot express. (Romans 8:26)*

I read in Mark, Chapter 9, how a man told Jesus that an evil spirit caused his son to go into dangerous convulsions that let his son fall into fires and onto the ground. He said the boy had been like that since childhood and that the apostles could not remove the evil spirit. Jesus asked to have the boy brought to Him. The father expressed some hesitation that Jesus could drive out the evil spirit. When Jesus told him that, *"Everything is possible to one who has faith." (Mark 9:23)*, he answered, *"I do believe, help my unbelief." (Mark 9:24*). And the demon was driven out of the boy. That one phrase became the MOST frequent small prayer that I uttered during my times of doubt—*help my unbelief, Lord.* Ask the Lord to help your unbelief. All things are possible. *When you call to me, when you go to pray to me, I will listen to you. (Jeremiah 29:12)*

Heavenly Pearls of Wisdom

Ignore clichés. Seek the truth for yourself and it will be revealed to you.

Claim your inheritance. God is anxious to give it to you.

Focus on and bless others. It lets God's grace flow through you and heals you and them.

Be grateful to God. Gratitude raises your energy vibrations and assists in healing.

Give up the heavy gluten. Our wheat is not what it used to be.

Breathe deeply. Make time for sessions, as your body craves the oxygen.

Read your Bible or other Holy Book. This is a time when you need inspiration.

5
Finding the Lord

July 4—Independence Day
"My grace is within you. Look for it—seek it—you have received grace to think differently, speak differently, to give stamina to your soul, and grace to strengthen your faith. Continue to pray for grace and mercy.

Each person I bring to you for a purpose. And 'what you do to the least of my brethren', applies to them also. Give grace to them. Receive them as you did Matthew."

Matthew, thank you for your sacrifice to protect our freedom, and for the Iraqi children.

When I heard the powerful words concerning other people, I spent the next 10 days listing in my journal every single person that I met or talked to that day—and I asked God to bless them. I didn't think that I encountered many people, but at the end of those days, the count stood at over 100! Even just to smile at the grocery clerk or the waiter/waitress affirms his or her life. We don't realize how powerful we are in the name of the Lord!

July 14
Today was Dustin and Angela's wedding reception. I had such a good time. I am so happy to be healed and with family. It

is good to see them healthy and happy. I am expecting even greater blessings on us all. I claim them dear Lord. Amen.

Expecting the Best—Hope

I visited Maggie at her home. She was having more trouble as a result of the chemotherapy. Her cancer cells had gotten immune to the chemotherapy, tumors were growing again, and another one was now growing in her brain. They were going to give her a new chemotherapy drug and brain surgery.

"Maggie, Maggie!" I begged. "Won't you please try some alternative treatments or medicine—anything—even something small to start—green tea, supplements, liver detoxification, juicing—anything?"

"No, I don't think I can do that."

"Why won't you at least TRY?"

"Because I don't want to have false hope."

"What is wrong with hope?"

"I've gotten my hopes up before and the let down is devastating. I just want to live long enough to see my son turn 18." (He was currently 16.)

Words escaped me. Here was hopelessness staring me in the face and I felt powerless. Her doctor had told her that she had maybe 24 months to live. He told her that chemo was the only hope she had of prolonging her life. What kind of hope was in that?

"I'm 8 months into this so I figure from what the doctors said that I've got 16 left." She believed this like it was a revelation from God.

"Maggie, don't give in to this. The doctor is not God! There is ALWAYS hope."

"Not for me."

I sadly shook my head and changed the subject. We said our good-byes. All the way home I pondered, "What is something I can give her that she might try—one small change she might make?" An idea came to me.

I brought her a jar of the Essiac tea that I brewed, along with instructions on how to take it. She said, "Thanks, Diana," and put it in the refrigerator. "You will try it, won't you?" I asked, hopefully.

"I don't want to take anything unless I check with the doctor," was her reply. A very sarcastic thought popped into my head. "Sure, the doctor who said you are dying—he's not going to sanction anything that might help you and prove him wrong." But, I said nothing. I wanted her to have hope and yet, I couldn't force it on her. It was frustrating. Upon inquiring a few weeks later, she revealed that she never asked him and never tried it. Sometimes, we have to accept that not everyone is able to receive or wants the help we so desperately want to give them. Her brain surgery was a success, but she was going to resume chemotherapy. I didn't know how she suffered through it. I prayed for her. I didn't know what to pray for exactly, so I asked the Lord to shower his love and kindness upon her.

> July 21
> Lord, what is my fear? Why am I so afraid? **"Your fear is that your will is not my will. Because your will is to help others and not just yourself, it is my will also. You are becoming. I took 32 years preparing. When the flower blooms, it will be a beautiful day. You are unfolding like a flower. I have great things planned for you on earth. You will help others. You will teach others. You ARE teaching them now. I work through you. All is well. All will come in good time. You cannot rush the unfolding of a flower."** Lord, forgive my impatience and frustration. *Therefore, submit to God. (James 4:7)*

What, exactly, is "false hope"? Is it a lack of faith? Is it a fear of having hope? Do we fear that the circumstances are overwhelming to the point that God can't help us? Is "false hope" placing our trust in something or someone other than God? There is always hope in the Lord, especially when we don't believe circumstances can change and don't 'see' anything happening or changing. I think the Bible says it best. *But hope that is seen is no hope at all. For who hopes for what he already has? (Roman 8:24).* It is best to make a conscious decision to choose life and tell the Lord our decision. I first became aware of that from listening to Michele at a meeting. She stated that we basically have two choices. We can stay at a lower level of unconsciousness and darkness that allows us just to let anyone do anything they want to us, even if it kills us. Or, we can rise to a higher level of consciousness and know that we have a choice. I told Michele that evening, "I didn't realize that I had a choice!" I had been mentally and spiritually stumbling around in the darkness. I had to make a choice and change would come. Then, once I made the choice, I had to place my hope in Him alone—not a doctor—not any human.

That doesn't mean that He doesn't guide us to a human or some other resource, but we are not to place our trust in that particular resource—only God. *But, if we hope for what we do not see, we eagerly wait for it with perseverance. (Romans 8:25)* I noticed that this passage does not say we fearfully wait. It says we <u>eagerly</u> wait for our hopes, which means we <u>expect</u> them. When we expect something, even if we don't see it yet, and feel the feelings of having it, it arrives. That is why, in my journal, my intention was to write and feel as if what I wanted had already appeared.

The best illustration, for me, is the movie *A Christmas Story* from 1983.[1] The main character, 9-year-old Ralphie, wanted a carbine action Red Ryder™ BB gun for Christmas. He told his mother and father over and over that he wanted it. He visualized using it. He hoped for it and expected it. His mom tried to discourage him by saying, "You'll shoot your eye out!" He wrote a paper about his desire for the gun in school and even the teacher, Mrs. Shields, wrote across his paper, "You'll shoot your eye out!" Then, he asked Santa for the BB gun and what did Santa say? "You'll shoot your eye out, kid!" But, nothing deterred his hope and expectation. On Christmas morning, just as he was about to give up hope with each non-Red Ryder-gun present he unwrapped, he received it as his last gift. Hope and expect. *For the vision still has its time, presses on to fulfillment and will not disappoint; if it delays, wait for it, for it will surely come, it will not be late.(Habakkuk 2:3)* Hope, expect, and then wait for what we wish to manifest.

July 26

"Continue to trust me. I will lay out the path before you. I know what you desire. It shall be yours. Remember, O flower, the bloom is still emerging— patience, patience, patience. Wait before the Lord. Remember, you will be a living testament to my power. You are still finding your way."

Release the Past

One of the things Maggie liked to do was to read books. We were both in the Italian Order (Sons of Italy), so I brought her Italian stories or books by Italian authors. I also slipped in one of Michele O'Donnell's books (She has written three of them). I called Maggie back to talk about the books. She said that her hands and feet were now numb (neuropathy) from the chemotherapy, so she could no longer cook, brush her hair or teeth, and could barely walk, but she could still read. We talked about the humor in the Italian stories and then I tiptoed gently into asking her about Michele's second book called *THE GOD WE'VE CREATED*[2]. Her statements burned permanently into my mind.

"Maggie, have you read the other book, the one by Michele?"

"I've read parts of it." I'm not so sure she did.

"Do you realize that it's not God's will for you to suffer and die?"

"Diana, I can't accept that. I've had a horrible past."

"God doesn't care about that. You're a wonderful secretary, wife, and mother. It's now that matters."

"You don't understand. I sinned so much and did some pretty terrible things when I was younger that I'm not proud of."

"Many of us have done sinful things. I could tell you some stories about myself, too."

"I don't deserve to be saved. I am suffering for what I did before."

"What can I do to convince you that God has forgiven you and does NOT want to see you suffer?"

She paused, sighed heavily and said sadly, "I don't know."

August 8

I have asked God so many times to let me help Maggie. I have received no audible answer, but I had a strange dream the other night. I was sitting at a desk and next to me was a gigantic vat of boiling oil. A cinnamon roll fell into the oil and sank deeper and deeper. I remember thinking that the poor cinnamon roll was going to get totally soaked with grease. I started to put my hand in to retrieve it, but I realized that if I did, my hand would be severely burned. So, I felt forced to sit and watch it become transformed into a greasy, hard, crusty, mess. What was the meaning of this dream? I prayed about it because it disturbed me. And the Lord gave me the answer.

He revealed to me that the cinnamon roll represents Maggie (because I often describe her as a very sweet person). The boiling oil represents the influences of thoughts she has internalized (that it is God's will that she suffer, or it is punishment for past sins), and belief in current medical treatments. She is "soaking up" these thoughts and beliefs. My hand beginning to reach in is my strong desire to help her, but she is already too far gone and too deeply immersed in erroneous beliefs. Any attempt on my part will have a detrimental effect on my own healing. I am being told to let her go. Lord, this is most difficult for me. The "whys" are not for me to ask or try to answer. From this moment forward, I will simply be her friend and pray for her.

I turned to my Bible for answers. I began to get a little frightened. Did I have it wrong? Did Michele's book get it wrong? Were we meant to suffer some more for past sins? Believe me, I was getting a little nervous. No cherub wings were coming out of my back. I, too, had sinned in the past. I felt a weakness creeping into my faith again. Was I totally forgiven? What did Jesus' death mean? Was it just something people said? I needed help now more than ever. After all, since I couldn't convince Maggie, was I truly convinced myself? *Do not fear, for I have redeemed you; I have called you by name; you are mine! When you pass through the waters, I will be with you; and through the rivers, they will not overflow you. When you walk through the fire, you will not be scorched, nor will the flame burn you. For I am the Lord your God... (Isaiah 43:1-3)*

> August 9
> **"My plan continues to unfold in you. ALL is forgiven. Forget the past. Dwell with me now. Here I am for you. Here is my MERCY.** *For I will be merciful to their iniquities, and I will remember their sins no more. (Hebrews 8:12)* **Partake of it gladly—bring Me to yourself. Think of Me often. I direct what you should do. Your trust is encouragement to Me. Great things, Diana, great things are possible. Do not rule anything out. Have faith. Be mine and mine alone. My Spirit is in you and I am beside you."**

After much prayer and introspection, to even think about the bad parts of the past serves absolutely no purpose, except to make people feel discouraged. What is the good in that? Nothing can be gained by it—the lesson from anything bad was learned long ago when it occurred. It behooves people to remain in the "now." I saw how devastating it was to focus on the bad things of the past. God reassured me that the past was not important and the following scriptural passages confirmed it as so. *It is I, I, who wipe out, for my own sake, your offenses; your sins I remember no more. Would you have me remember, have us come to trial? (Isaiah 43:25)* No trial for me, God. I'm glad you choose not to remember. Help me to forget also. I noticed He did NOT say, "You'd better watch out. I might reconsider forgiving you after you've repented and I will inflict a new punishment on you." What He did say was, *I have brushed away your offenses like a cloud, your sins like a mist; return to me, for I have redeemed you. (Isaiah 44:22)* Humans aren't able to heal if those guilty, self-deprecating, "I-haven't-paid-enough-yet-for-my-past-sins" thoughts are allowed to fester. We are paid up. Let them go.

Getting rid of past guilt and shame took practice for me. Every time any thought of some error I'd committed in the past tried to eat at me, I stated out loud, "Be gone from me, you evil thoughts! I have repented and **know** the Lord has forgiven me and forgotten about it. You cannot get me with that. Be gone in the name of Jesus the Christ! He is the one true Lord and Savior!" And the thoughts of guilt or shame left me. I did it often and still do. We have plenty to deal with today, on which we focus. That is enough.

> August 16
> Lord, I hope that my prayers are enough. Maybe I should spend more time praying—more hours. **"Long periods with me are not required. Quality time with me is. I am revealing myself slowly to you just as I do to others who seek me. Watch for it—be alert—it comes in a breath."**
>
> Am I doing enough for others? What should I do? **"Man does not understand that goodness flows. It is not a see saw—you do something good for me, and I do something good for you. It is better to do good for those who cannot repay. Let my goodness flow."**

Healing with Foods

A friend asked me, "Since you are on such a strict eating plan, what CAN you eat?"

"Well, for breakfast, I eat a bowl of rice or corn cereal, with either soy, almond, goat, or rice milk. With that I eat half of an apple or a banana. I make a cup of herbal coffee such as Tecchino™."

"Can you have eggs?"

"Yes, eggs with spelt toast but no bacon! And some mornings, I eat gluten-free frozen waffles with some sort of protein."

"What about lunch?"

"I eat mostly salads or sandwiches made with tuna or nitrite-free deli turkey or chicken. I also don't mind boiled eggs. I look for organic vegetables and buy spelt bread for the sandwiches. I buy baked potato chips. It's really not so bad. But, I don't eat iceberg lettuce—only dark greens like romaine or spinach. On my salad, I use olive oil and a dash of Celtic sea salt."

"You know, it really does sound doable. When you told us all of the stuff you couldn't eat, I didn't think anything was left!"

"I miss cheese the most. I love cheese. In fact, before all of this happened, I absolutely craved cheese and ate quite a bit of it. I thought it would be good for me, but I was actually contributing more to the problem. Dinner is a little tougher. I don't always cook so I have to modify some. I might pick up a cooked roasted chicken. Then, I just cook up a vegetable or two to have with it. Sweet potatoes and baked potatoes are OK, too. And I have a piece of spelt bread or a spelt breadstick."

"What other dinners do you have?"

"Cooked spelt spaghetti with browned ground turkey in my own tomato sauce is my favorite! Or Lloyd will grill turkey sausages on the grill—yum, yum! We also make our own pizza with spelt crust, vegetables, browned ground turkey, and goat cheese. Goat cheese tastes sort of like Feta cheese and I like the taste of it. I never thought I'd be eating things like that either. I'm still investigating new recipes for good salmon and fish, to be creative."

"And what do you drink?"

"The hardest part was giving up iced tea. I used to go to Luby's Cafeteria® and drink at least 3 glasses. Now, I drink distilled water.

No sodas—not even diet—since they contain phosphorus and remove calcium from your bones. Distilled water has all of the impurities removed. I also drink Japanese powdered green tea called Sencha or Matcha. I order it online."

"I've heard of Chinese green tea, but how did you discover Japanese green tea?"

"Lloyd and I went to Florida. When we arrived, I asked the hotel concierge to direct us to a healthy restaurant, one that the locals frequented. We were eating there and noticed everyone drinking this iced green drink. The owner, Simon, told us about Japanese green tea and how beneficial it was for all sorts of illnesses and conditions. Many of the local doctors in the area send their patients to Simon for his advice. When I asked him about people with cancer, he very enthusiastically endorsed it for their return to health. I asked him how much one should have and his reply was, 'As much as they can drink!' "

"Do you feel like this eating plan is helping?"

"I feel like my body is changing slowly from the inside out—being reworked. I heard that every 120 days, you make new cells and old ones die. So, I don't know how many cells I have, but I'm giving my body new fuel to build healthy ones and kick out those that are unhealthy. I figure in a short while, I'll have a brand new body and I feel GREAT! Slowly but surely, the discipline of eating and drinking correctly will pay off."

"I don't know if I could make all of those changes."

"My best advice is, if you are not ill, to make one change at a time. Visit the health food store and discover the new array of foods available to you that are much healthier than what most of America eats."

"You know, I can do that. I think I'll start by trying to eliminate regular iced tea. I drink too much iced tea."

"Good for you! Your body will thank you in many ways and let me know if I can help." *No discipline seems pleasant at the time, but painful. Later on, however, it produces a harvest of righteousness and peace for those who have been trained by it. Therefore, strengthen your feeble arms and weak knees. (Hebrews 12:11-12)*

August 25
"Continue to be patient. You are doing better. I am turning you slowly like a large ship on the sea. I am gently setting the path for you. I am bending you gently. To change directions abruptly is not easy for a large ship. Likewise, to change directions abruptly is not good for the soul. Be patient as I work all for your good." Thank you, Lord. Thank you for all of your abundance and goodness. I am open to change and I gladly embrace and accept it.

August 28
"Your consciousness is tuned into the heavenly voice. That voice serves you well. Other voices can be like clanging cymbals. The heavenly voice brings peace. It is kind. Listen to it often. I speak constantly to you in many ways. Sometimes, you are listening and sometimes, you are preoccupied. You will always know my word. Impart it to others."

August 29
"Part of man's challenge is the search for me—the longing—I have placed it in his heart. I am here but he must find me. He must discover his relationship with me just as you are doing. I am one with man but he chooses to separate from me. Then, after the suffering of separation, he wishes to come back! For man does not always appreciate what is easily given." *O, satisfy us early with your mercy, that we may rejoice and be glad all our days. (Psalm 90:11)*

According to Donald Yance, a certified nutritionist and clinical master herbalist, in his book entitled *HERBAL MEDICINE, HEALING, AND CANCER*[3], nutrition, diet, and herbs are essential to healing. It is critical that we add foods or drinks to our diet that accomplish one or more of the following: 1) detoxifying the liver, 2) inhibiting tumor formation, and 3) boosting the immune system. For example, he states that green tea inhibits tumor initiation, helps the liver detoxify, and blocks abnormal cell growth. He further explains that researchers continue to find that those who eat the most vegetables and fruits have the lowest rates of cancer.

The list of foods that are beneficial is quite extensive. He recommends one or two servings (1/2 cup) of carotene rich vegetables, such as carrots, yams, squash, pumpkin, tomatoes, melons and dark greens every day. He also encourages one serving of cruciferous vegetables—MUST be COOKED—every day. These include cabbage, broccoli, Brussels sprouts, cauliflower, and radishes. Asparagus is another vegetable with anticancer ingredients; it must also be cooked. These foods, if eaten raw, contain ingredients that suppress the thyroid. Cancer patients often have a low functioning thyroid and aren't aware of it.

I refer the reader to any number of books written on the benefits of many of the vegetables. Eat those organic vegetables! Our moms were right when they encouraged us to eat our veggies!

September 9

Another month has gone by and I am more convinced than ever that God, through Jesus, has had mercy and healed me. I know his truth. I used to dream that I could fly and then one day, the dreams stopped. Now, I had a dream that I flapped my arms and I flew! Hallelujah! I fly again! I felt so light and it was wonderful! Thank you, Lord! I think this is symbolic—my life is taking flight! Up, up, and away! I love you, Jesus!

Heavenly Pearls of Wisdom

Release the Past. Your past doesn't matter, only now matters.
Eat dark green vegetables. Include broccoli and asparagus.
Expect the best. The Lord wants to give it to you.
Brief prayers <u>are</u> heard. Prayers don't have to be long and wordy. God hears even a one word prayer—"help."

6
Fullness of Grace

Sept 21
We found out that the back part of the foundation of our home has sunk. We hope to have it repaired by the warranty company and/or builder. We are told to look for symbolic meanings in situations we encounter in life. So, what words did I hear from the Lord today? **"As you read my word, you will speak my word with wisdom. I am laying the foundation in you—preparing you for works. Know me. Know my way. Keep reading of me. Bind your mind to mine. I show the way but many do not follow. They choose their own way and when it becomes thorny, they fall and are confused. You see the way and are proceeding along it. Continue—I am always here to guide you. ASK."** Oh, Lord, thank you for the guidance. It is so much easier when I turn all over to you. And I am so thankful that you want us to ask you for what we desire. I know that, at times, we try to solve our own problems. We forget to simply ask you. I need your help with the house foundation and I pray for a solid spiritual foundation as well.

Symbolic Meanings

Lloyd and I planned on putting in wood flooring back in November before everything fell apart for me healthwise a few months later. I was excited about the thought of getting rid of the old worn carpet. But, some of our doors wouldn't stay closed and others wouldn't stay open. This was a warning that a potential problem existed. We hired an engineer to evaluate the foundation and he gave us a report. When he finished his examination, I eagerly asked him, "So, how is our foundation doing? Is everything OK?" He hesitated and then replied in a serious tone, "No, ma'am, everything is not ok."

"What's the matter?"

"Your foundation has sunk over four inches."

"FOUR inches?"

"Yes, all along the back part of the house."

"That's quite a bit. Why aren't there any cracks in the house?"

"You DO have some small cracks beginning to form in the sheetrock. And your entire house is tilting backwards. That's why your house foundation pulled away from the driveway and left a gap in front."

"Oh, no! I can't believe it! Are you sure?" (I always asked anyone that when I didn't quite believe what I'd just heard. It's a habit of mine, I'm told.)

"Yes, ma'am, I'm sure."

"Well, what do we do now?"

"You'll have to have the foundation repaired."

"You mean I can't have wood flooring installed?" I knew the answer to that. I guess I had to hear him say it aloud.

"You could, but when you have the foundation repaired, it will probably cause the wood to buckle."

"About how much does it cost to repair a foundation?"

"Well, I don't actually repair foundations. But the companies I have done evaluations for charge anywhere from $20,000 to $40,000, depending on what method you use."

"Heaven forbid! We don't have that kind of money to spare! What shall I do?" Tears welled up in my eyes at this point.

"How old is this house?"

"Nine years old" I said through tears. We had been so happy to have a brand new house back then and now THIS!

"Do you have a 10-year home warranty?"

"Yes, we sure do!"

"You need to call the warranty company and file a claim."

"How long does THAT take?" I said, tears now streaming down my face. This was disappointing. The foundation had to be repaired or no one would ever buy the house when we decided to sell. Or, if they did buy it, the price would be ridiculously low. As a real estate agent, I'd seen it happen and knew the results.

It was now 10 months later and we were still trying to get resolution to this problem. No wood floors were in the immediate future. However, it seems that all the unusual things that happen to us are symbolic of what is going on in our inner life.

Someone asked me, "Did things in the Old Testament happen as the Bible says or were they just symbolic?" My answer was, "They did actually happen AND they were also symbolic." She said, "I never thought of it as being BOTH. That is most interesting." The same thing holds true for our lives. Things do happen to us and they are symbolic.

In this case, the foundation of my faith and trust needed repair. I guess my warranty company (God) agreed to heal me in more than just the physical sense. I needed spiritual healing as well. I needed a new foundation upon which to build spiritual truths and experiences.

We carry with us, in our being, every memory of past events, which we have categorized as "good memories" or "bad memories." If they are not in one of those two categories, we usually don't remember them. Some of those memories include events which shaped our spiritual opinions about situations, God, ourselves, or others. The body is not what needs healing. It is the soul that is wounded and the body is reflecting that. The soul is what needs healing and only God is capable of healing the soul. When the body alone is treated, it is the proverbial placing of a bandage over the wound and ignoring the underlying cause. God was tearing down my old opinions and beliefs, right down to the foundation. The foundation was being leveled, and soon, the rebuilding of the spiritual "house" would take place. The healing of the spirit was taking place.

> October 24
> I was sitting and relaxing when the Lord spoke these words, **"I fill your being when you make space for me. I flow through you when you allow me to. I am the God of justice and righteousness but I am also the God of mercy and tenderness. Remember that."** At that moment, for some reason, my whole being felt a fullness that I cannot describe accurately. My heart was bursting with love and gratitude. I began to cry and thank the Lord. As I was sobbing, I heard him speak further. **"Now you feel me as you have asked. Your heart is my heart. Let our hearts rest together. I am working all things in you and through you. You are serving me and will serve me more. I will ignite the passion in you. You have felt my presence. Your power comes from me. If you have no power, it is because you don't believe. Your hidden talent, that you have asked me to reveal to you is this—the power to heal others in many ways. Learn from me. Use it—do not be afraid. It is not you but me that worketh these things. Rely on me. Call on me. Accept this gift."**
>
> Lord, I am overwhelmed. I accept your gifts—teach me how and when to use them wisely. May I remain humble and only do all for your glory. Amen.

Remembering to Ask

The lesson that I constantly work on is remembering to ASK. When anything other than peace and contentment is felt, asking the Lord for help is required. When I am afraid, I ask the Lord to give me courage. During times that I am angry, I ask the Lord to replace that anger with grace. When I am doubtful, I ask Him to increase my belief.

One day, I asked the Lord to let me feel his presence. I told Him that I believed in Him but that, just once, I needed to FEEL Him. And He answered. I asked Him to reveal any hidden talents that I could use to serve Him or which of my current talents to use. And He answered. I asked Him to heal me spiritually, mentally, and physically. His answer continues to unfold to this day.

October 30
I am continuing my holistic program. I know that my body has already changed drastically. I am so thankful that my symptoms are going away. My blood work is showing improvement. The clinic is very encouraging and it helps me that my friends and relatives are supportive. The memory of this is beginning to seem like a bad dream that never happened.

I read part of the old and new testaments in the Bible every day before my day starts. **"Remember my words. My words will see you and others through much. Believe in me. I cannot stress that enough. Weak hearts can be forever lost. It is I who has the power to strengthen, especially if asked. ASK. Continue to ask. I never grow weary of listening. It is man who tires of asking. I hear and obey the command for help. I hear all people, even those who think that they are insignificant. You have heard and accepted. I am pleased."** Lord, I always wish to please you, but how do I know if what I do, don't do, or think, is not pleasing to you? **"Listen to the conscience I have given you. It will tell you when something is not pleasing to me. You will also know because you will not be at peace."** *A man's conscience can tell him his situation better than seven watchmen in a lofty tower. Most important, pray to God, to set your feet in the path of truth. (Sirach 37:14-15)* Thank you for all that you reveal to me. I am going to continue to ask and encourage others to ask also. Help me to always remember to ask and to know what to ask FOR. Amen.

I never thought to ask God to speak to me, yet he did and still does. If that is what your heart seeks, I recommend that you ask Him to speak to you. However, in so doing, it is wise to "make space for Him," by seeking some quiet time. A friend asked me, "How do you find the quiet time?" I reminded her that, in the beginning, I spent much time in the restroom. I have an entire library in there. I should have had Lloyd build book shelves. Soaking 20-minute baths were also required with a detoxifying agent added to the water. I used that time to speak to the Lord and reflect. Everyday, I set aside some time for reading my Bible, prayer, and silence. I still talk to Him in the shower, any time that I am by myself. We have been under drought conditions the past 2 years. When I am outside hand watering the yard with the hose (since we often get put on water restrictions), it's the perfect time to converse with God. Ask Him to help you find the quiet time with Him. Once again, it is holy to ask for EVERY LITTLE THING. Even a small prayer is your communication with God. You may say something as simple as, "Lord, thank you for the beautiful butterfly I just saw," or "Lord, give me peace even though I want to argue."

Some people are afraid to ask the Lord to reveal Himself to them. They fear that He will ask them to give up all of their possessions, become a missionary, or some other drastic change. Do not fear. He will lead you gently to anything new and will prepare the way. It will all unfold naturally and give you passion for the endeavor. You may already have a passion, but don't know how to fulfill your desire.

God will not compete with the "noise" that surrounds us. He is too polite. Most of us have a radio on constantly, are watching television, playing video games, talking on our cell phones, reading e-mail, listening to the music on our electronic devices, texting, running our kids or grandkids all over the country, or talking to our friends and family. We have taken up all of the "spiritual space" with other noise. That is why we long for some time in the woods, or near the ocean, with no internet, no cell phone. Our hearts are longing for that time to hear God. Ask and make time to listen. He desires to talk to you on God's cell phone!

December 24, Christmas Eve Early
I returned yesterday from a flight to Iowa for my Godmother aunt Philipa's (Phyllis) funeral. We call that Gumare (goo mar' ay) in Italian dialect. She was 89 and I loved her dearly. I still have the Bulova watch she bought me for my high school graduation over 40 years ago, even though it has long since quit ticking.

My cousin Lucia (her daughter) and I were talking after the funeral service and I touched her arm to console her as we finished viewing some pictures of my aunt. She immediately looked at me with a startled expression and started to walk away. Then she turned and said to me, "<u>You</u> have the power to heal others.....I felt it when you touched me." I freaked out because I had received that message in prayer. I had told NO one...how did she know? I cried because it confirmed what I had heard but I was also scared that I didn't know HOW to heal people! Lucia, who is very in tune with the Spirit, informed me that it is not me doing the healing... it is the Lord. I am so lost in the category of healing others. The Lord's got some work to do!!

Christmas Eve Late
I received a call today from my dad that my mom has been rushed to the hospital with a stroke. I am praying and sending as much grace, healing, and wholeness as the Lord will allow to flow through me. I wish I could be there, but trying to get a flight is going to be impossible. My dad is beside himself. Jesus, have mercy. In your name, O Jesus, I banish the darkness from my mother and fill in that gap with mercy, grace, and the light of God. Fear gripped my heart and I prayed.

I talked to Melissa when I went for a clinic appointment and cried that I could not be in the hospital to lay hands on my mother. She reminded me that in the spirit world, there is no distance between spirits, that I could help heal her from right where I was. That helped me tremendously.

Christmas Eve Midnight
Dad called and mom is doing better. She stopped vomiting and is coherent, even though her speech is still slurred. Thank you, Jesus. I will continue to send her healing and prayer until I am able to fall asleep.

December 25 Christmas Day
My sister Joann was able to drive up to Iowa from Kansas to be with dad. My deaf brother showed her where all of the food was that my mom had purchased to cook for Christmas dinner. She put it all together and made a wonderful meal. Then, they took the meal up to the hospital for my mom. Now that is true love. I am there in spirit.

Mom is almost back to normal!!! Hallelujah! Thank you, Lord, for hearing our prayers! I see her as whole, perfect, and complete! What a magical Christmas this is.

Dec 26th
Mom went home from the hospital today. Yea! I know that my dad is extremely happy and so thankful. She will need some physical therapy for a few weeks for the right side of her body. O, Lord, I claim total recovery for her. I trust you. Amen.

No Distance Too Great

My spiritual lessons continue. But, to me, the most important one here is that we do not have to be physically in each other's presence to pray for them or to affect what happens to them. We can pray and heal and send grace from afar because our spirit is capable of being there. God fills in any gaps. There is a part in the Bible in which the Roman soldier approached Jesus. *And when Jesus entered Capernaum, a centurion came to him, imploring him, and saying, 'Lord, my servant is lying paralyzed at home, fearfully tormented.' Jesus said to him, 'I will come and heal him.' But the centurion said, 'Lord, I am not worthy for you to come under my roof, but just say the word, and my servant will be healed.' And Jesus said to the centurion, 'Go; it shall be done for you as you have believed.' And the servant was healed that very moment. (Matt. 8:5-13)*

This passage is so powerful and all of us would do well to heed its importance. We CAN pray for others and believe that something good will happen across all time and space. St. Matthew's account gives confirmation of both precepts. We are all connected in some way and have a stronger connection with certain people than we do with others. That explains why mothers can feel when things are not right with one of their children who may live in another state or country. You can send grace and healing to others no matter where you are. And, at this very moment, there are people sending love, grace and healing to you, and I am one of them. Accept it gratefully. There is no distance between us.

January 5

A new year has begun, which I am most grateful to be here for, and the Lord spoke to me today saying, **"I know you wait patiently and sometimes you wonder. Do you doubt me?"** Lord, I feel that I am not worthy of all of your blessings or being healed. **"No one, of themselves, is worthy. But, I am in all people and things so how can they then NOT be worthy? Believe—all good things come to you. You know not from whence it comes, but it comes, as I am the Lord, thy God. All is possible for me beyond your expectations. It shall pour forth upon you until your heart wants to burst. Then, you must choose wisely and ask for my direction as you do**

now. Always remember, seek me. I am here but you must always seek me. I shall move you to do what is necessary for you and others. All is set in motion. My laws are immutable (unchangeable) just as I am." But, Lord, I am no one. I'm not renowned or known publicly in any way. I'm not a celebrity or politician. I am unknown. **"That is why I choose you—it is always the little ones that I choose for they are more pure of heart. Public figures are often already corrupted."** But, Father, you can accomplish anything and don't need me. **"It is <u>my</u> choice. I, too, choose. I sent my son, Jesus, to manifest my mercy upon all. I chose this also."**

January 16
It has been a year since the diagnosis was given to me. Notice that I did not say "my" disease or illness. I do not take ownership of it…it is not part of me. In fact, I'm sure that it is gone. I simply await visible proof. That is hard when you can't look inside yourself, but in a way, I'm thankful that I can't. Seeing something would only serve to try to frighten me. My pledge is to continue with the program and to focus on God and others. I only want to continue to do what is pleasing to the Lord. Nothing else is as important. **"My way is simple but not easy."** Lord, I know that you are correct. You only gave us two main commandments—to love God with our whole heart, mind, strength, and soul, and to love our neighbor as ourselves—DEFINITELY not easy! (The neighbor part.) **"Continue to bless others and heal. That is my will. All the day long it can be done—in my name. It is pleasing to me. Then, you use the power you have claimed—continue to claim and use it. Use it for your neighbor to show my love. Bless all that you come in contact with—even those you don't meet but only hear of. Bless your leaders for they need it much worse than ordinary men and women. They are in great peril. The devil roams freely among them and finds many weaknesses, such as greed for earthly power and money, upon which to feed.**

Pray—as much as possible. That, too, is my will. It can be accomplished anywhere, anytime, with great benefit. Prayer crosses all time and distance barriers. It is carried to heaven instantly. It has a purpose. It is never unheard. All petitions are answered in different ways. Always remain steadfast and it shall be manifested." Lord, please remain as the God of our country, no matter what you may hear from others. I ask you. *You shall be my people, and I will be your God. (Jeremiah 30:22)*

Our Leaders and Prayers

For our kings, our LEADERS, our priests and our fathers have not kept your law or paid attention to your commandments and your admonitions with which you have admonished them. But they, in their own kingdom, with your great goodness which you gave them, with the broad and rich land you set before them, did not serve you or turn from their evil deeds. (Nehemiah 9:34-35)

The Lord's messages made me wonder what else I should learn from God's words in the Bible. For me, the message was that each one of us must not rely on some government official to help us with health, wellness, money, or love. Many of them are not at all interested in us, but only in furthering their own "weaknesses." Politicians may start off with lofty goals but eventually, for many of them, the main goal becomes to get re-elected, and thus begins the moral downfall. With God, the most wondrous things can be accomplished that politicians and celebrities fail to achieve. Hard to imagine that we are that powerful, isn't it? We are connected to the Divine, one and only God. It is good to pray for our leaders that they will make divinely inspired choices in their lawmaking and in spending our money. *Do not be called leaders; for One is your leader, that is, Christ. (Matthew 23:10)*

I had bemoaned the fact that my holistic treatments were costing money and that it wasn't covered by insurance. What good was that line of thinking? I need to rely on God, not insurance. He has always taken care of me when insurance and the government did not. People were still coming to me for real estate and I asked the Lord to just continue to bring me resources as I needed them, which he continues to do. But, I believed that he would. Do I have doubtful moments or days about everything? Absolutely yes! And when I do, I ask the Lord to take those away and replace them with the belief and hope in Him. This is a constant movement. I take three steps forward and one step backward. It is part of climbing the mountain of faith.

January 26
"Your time is coming, Diana. Time to do great works. Here am I to guide you. What wonders will occur if you believe. All things are possible and I mean ALL things—even those that seem impossible. You have been given insight. I give you my grace. Let it flow. You are getting better at turning to me.

Many people do not think of me even once during the day. They are too caught up in the world. Stop—just stop—talk to me—ask me—feel me. I am here always. Blessed are those who seek my truth. For it does not come easy amidst so much deception in the world. I love all but am offended by many. Those who believe the truth are mine."

January 27
Today, the Lord spoke to me as I became calm. It is hard when the mind is not calm. **"Peace—be at peace—exterior and interior peace. Other souls can perceive the interior peace that I give freely. That is one of the attributes of the Heavenly Kingdom—peace. A peaceful heart is capable of much. It handles all with ease. It frets not for it knows from where all help comes, if and when needed. It asks. It believes and it receives—but in peace—not in worry.**

Parents want the child to look to them for everything. You

are spiritual children—maturing and growing—in need of guidance. When a child forgoes guidance and attempts tasks on its own, trouble follows. Blessed be those who seek my guidance. You are never alone. Amen." *Go in peace and may the Lord go before you. (Judith 8:35)*

February 9
Some days I believe that I am healed, other days I think I am improving, and other days I wonder if anything is happening at all. But, the Lord said, **"You are complete, whole, and perfect and soon you will have proof, proof of my glory. You still have work to do. You ARE a healer. Take on your role. I will lead you. I know what you need. I HAVE probed your heart. You will continue to serve me. There will be no more muddiness or uncertainty. You will be certain. It shall unfold. All is in readiness. Why do you think that I direct you to certain scriptures? Because they apply. They are your bread, fed to you by me. I feed my sheep and they know me. Amen."**

February 11
O, Lord, the waiting is SO hard—waiting for all that you have promised—the outward proof of my healing and your glory, the assignment you have for me. I DO believe and am SO grateful, but I am impatient—waiting for you to walk out to me on the water as I sit in my boat, trying not to paddle frantically. I trust you, Jesus. Amen.

February 13
It struck me that today is the 13th. Some people consider this number unlucky, but I feel blessed. Since the apostles replaced Judas, who betrayed Jesus and then hung himself, with Matthias, there were 12 apostles and I am a disciple too. That makes me number 13. I am the 13th. *I will praise you with my whole heart; In the day when I cried out, you answered me. (Psalm 138:1,3)*

While in prayer, the Lord said, **"I am bringing all things to you. It IS my divine hand. Your mind is quiet and ready to receive me and I AM here—not a figment of your imagination as you fear, but really HERE. I speak gently but with conviction. Do NOT filter my words—take them as they are—as they come. All good things are yours—believe—soon your heart will burst with excitement. What you long for comes true. You are in the 'positive plane.' "**

February 26

Every year, the Living Beyond Disease ministry puts on a weekend retreat, lead by Michele Longo O'Donnell. Lloyd and I attended. It was quite uplifting and I gained more knowledge and wisdom in the spiritual realm. No business conducted, no phones, just absorbing.

The Lord later said to me, **"I am all that you need. Look to me for all. Do not look elsewhere. Trust ME. I prepare the way. It will be effortless, fun, and exciting. There are so many needy souls for what you will provide. What they receive will be so great that they will be grateful. It is of me—it is good. Trust me—be patient. All is in readiness and I bring it to you. I place the desire in your heart as a way of glorifying me."** Lord, I am eager and humbly willing to follow where you lead me. I know that my life is not my own, but yours completely. Amen.

Patience is Difficult

As I re-read my journal, I realized how many times the Lord had to tell me to have patience. I knew one could pray for patience, but I always applied it to the times when I was impatient with my children or my husband–not to situations in my life or healing. It is difficult to believe in what we hope for all of the time but, once one believes, it is even more difficult to be patient and wait upon the Lord. In this society, we want to take a pill or drink a magic liquid and have our problem disappear instantly. We want a pill to lose weight, a magic elixir to kill cancer, and a mystical potion to heal our mental wounds. If God gave us everything immediately, we would be like spoiled children who wanted everything now, missing the lessons along the way.

The movie, *WILLY WONKA AND THE CHOCOLATE FACTORY*, comes to mind. If you have seen the movie, do you recall how annoying Augustus was when he demanded everything right now? And the little girl Violet that popped the flavor-changing gum into her mouth, because she didn't want to wait until Mr. Wonka had perfected it—and when the blueberry flavor came, she turned blue and her whole body became swollen[1]. All because of her impatience.

Patience—it sounds so trite and yet it is so important. I wanted to be healed, finished with any form of treatment, have plenty of money, and I wanted it NOW. When I became impatient...what was the answer? I prayed for patience—of course. But, the days still went by just as slowly, with improvement seen and felt little by little. I took comfort in that fact that even Jeremiah, the famous prophet in the Bible, had to wait for days at a time to receive an answer from God. Some army officers asked Jeremiah, *Pray that the Lord your God will tell us where we should go and what we should do. "I have heard you," said Jeremiah the prophet. "I will certainly pray to the Lord your God, as you have requested" (Jeremiah 42:3-4)* He never seemed to reproach God for taking so long in earth terms, but simply asked God and waited for the answer. *Ten days later the word of the Lord came to Jeremiah. (Jeremiah 42:7)* Can you imagine having to wait ten days when we are used to instant messaging? It's like torture. Ah, sweet patience.

Have you ever cut yourself and then watched how slowly the wound heals? Even a small one takes at least a good week to become ordinary skin again with some scarring. The laws of nature dictate that all things have a season and a time, including healing. Why aren't we healed quickly? Some people are and some are not...each according to his need. Apparently, I needed to learn patience and a few other lessons too. *There is an appointed time for everything. And there is an appointed time for every event under heaven...He has made everything appropriate in its time... (Ecclesiastes 3:1,11)*

March 2

Today, this was spoken to me, **"Prepare yourself. Continue to read, study, practice, and impart my word. I will send you the Holy Spirit to put the words in your mouth. You are of me. It is I who speaks to you. Do not doubt. There is work for you to do. You ARE one of my disciples now and forever. In a little while, things will come to pass and you will marvel at my goodness and delight in me. I am your Lord. There is no other.**

I am the right hand AND the left hand. You are the instrument. I am shaping you so that my hands fit comfortably on the instrument. You are an instrument of my peace, love, joy, and healing. You are healed so that you may help others heal. I will send you the necessary resources. It has begun. Amen."

Every day seemed to bring some answers and yet more questions. What did he have in mind for me? Only time, patience, and trust would tell. I hoped I was ready but then, I trusted that God wouldn't "send" me until it was the appointed time. Where was I going? Life is such a mystery.

Heavenly Pearls of Wisdom

Look for symbolic meanings. What is manifested in your outer world is often a reflection of what needs to be "fixed" in your inner world.

Ask God for every little thing. He wants you to.

Grace can be sent from afar. You can be the sender or the receiver.

Pray for our leaders. But don't rely on them for your needs. Only God supplies what you need and in ways you never expect. Leaders cannot heal you.

Pray for interior peace. It's not just a hippie term. We need it to connect with God and to heal. If you aren't at peace, you won't heal.

Ask for patience. Patience to believe that which you do not yet see, patience to wait for the good things you claim, and patience for the Lord to lead you.

7
God's Grace Flows

March 22
Today in prayer the Lord said, **"Continue to believe. Your belief is getting stronger and with it, the fulfillment of your desires. We are in harmony. This is why you feel peace. Great things are yours—claim them—continue to claim and they appear. There is nothing that my father cannot do. Resurrect your mind. Think all and it appears.**

Love is the key. People do not understand this. 'How can love bring what we desire?' they say. Love is the fulfillment of all. Those who truly love accomplish great things and attract others to help them. You are doing so. Use your love and light. It comes from me. My hand is over all. Great things are forming in my universe for you—great things—more than you can imagine on earth. There are many rewards, on earth and in heaven, and you shall partake of them. You shall have your proof. Just as my resurrection was my proof to all of the truth of my words to them, your resurrection is at hand. Oh, Glory in me—glory in me and with me. You ARE my disciple. I expect great things in return. They will continue to be revealed to you.

All roads are being paved. The gold is under your feet as you walk the golden path. The work I have for you has many

facets like a diamond, each contributing to its brilliance. Love will guide you through all. You are mine—joy in that—bring joy to all."

March 28

I have fears again, for some reason. I am experiencing some doubt that I am being healed. Why have these thoughts tried to stay with me? I still don't have visible proof of being healed yet. What is going on? In prayer, as if in answer, I heard, **"Do not doubt, Diana. All things take time to unfold according to my plan for you. Put aside impatience. Remember, you cannot rush the unfolding of a flower. You are the flower and all you do is the nectar, drawing others to yourself and me. Seek and you shall find. Fulfill my purpose as it is revealed each and every day. Pray—pray much—with every beat of your heart, for others and for yourself. I guide your thoughts. You do not need specifics yet. You are healing the remainder of your body. When it is complete, the work begins. You must have the strength to accomplish what I have set for you.** *I have heard your prayer; I have seen your tears... (Isaiah 38:5)*

You are to heal. You are a healer first and foremost. You have the power. Believe. Ask another, 'Do you wish to be healed?' Only if they answer yes do you proceed. Invoke me and the power of the kingdom—the power of the Holy Spirit. Ask for the keys. Some spirits are weary, weighed down with the burdens of guilt and perceived troubles. I gladly shoulder their burdens if they only ask. When they are free of the burdens, they are able to heal—physically, mentally and spiritually. Help them give the burdens to me. Amen."

April 2

I received a call from Maggie's sister. She called to tell me that Maggie passed away in the evening. I am so sad for the family and for her, that she allowed so much to be done to her—all to no avail. She had chemotherapy, more chemotherapy, different chemotherapy, brain surgery, more chemotherapy, a breathing machine, suffered much, and when she was too weak to walk, a chair that lifted her to a standing position. I went over to her house, visited, and we played with the chair. Her bed had been moved from upstairs down into the dining room because she was too weak to climb the stairs. I knew that she didn't look good, her entire body was swollen as well as her face, but I never thought she would die only one week after I had visited and she got that nifty chair. I did all that I could, but it wasn't enough to change the outcome. I feel weak—weak in faith, weak of heart. God told me I'm a healer and yet, I couldn't heal her.

I walked by a gigantic old oak tree and the tree seemed to tell me this story. "I have not always been so steadfast and strong. At one time, as a young tree, strong winds would come and bend me over sideways so badly that I thought I would surely break. Rain would fall so heavily that I would droop severely under the weight. But, every time, the sun would shine and the winds would be calm, and my life process would flourish. I grew taller and stronger and my roots became deeper to hold me fast. Now, I stand my ground, not to be moved."

Maggie, you were bent to the breaking point, you drooped under the weight of it all. But, the face of God has shown upon you. Now, you stand tall and steadfast in Him in the Heavenly kingdom, never to be moved. Thank you, God, for this wonderful friend and person. May you be with her grieving family and tell her that I am grateful for her friendship and all she did for me and that I love her. Amen.

Courage to Heal

Some kind of disciple I was turning out to be. Who can blame the 12 apostles for being skittish about preaching among the people? Who can blame them for asking Jesus why they couldn't always heal others? I had experienced my first death of a friend from cancer and it was devastating. Did I possess the courage to let God heal me slowly? Did I have the courage to help heal others—even if only with a kind word? I was frightened and apprehensive about my own healing and yet He told me I would heal others.

It was exciting to think I could heal others! People are under the mistaken impression that the ability to heal disappeared when the twelve apostles left this earth. Not so! One example is the conversion of Saul who was persecuting Christians long after the death of Jesus. He had been present when they stoned St. Stephen to death. He was knocked off of his horse suddenly one day and blinded by a bright light. Jesus spoke to him and said, *"Saul! Saul! Why do you persecute me?" (Acts 22:7)* Saul became blind from that moment on and had to be helped by his companions. But, Jesus commanded him to go to Damascus and ask for Ananias. He went to Damascus and found the man. *He stood beside me and said, 'Brother Saul, receive your sight!' And at that very moment, I was able to see him. (Acts 22:13)* And Saul's name was changed to Paul who became a zealous apostle of Christ. Ananias was not one of the original 12 apostles and yet he had the power to heal. Did we lose the power to heal? No! We lost the belief that we could heal. *Amen, amen I say to you, whoever believes in me will do the works that I do, and will do greater ones than these, because I am going to the Father. (John 14:12)*

God had shaken me to the core and said I should heal. Alas! How was I to go about it? Was I to walk up to any of my sick acquaintances or relatives and ask them if they want to be healed? I'm glad God said I wasn't ready yet. My time had not yet come. I thought of myself as a "healer in training".

Therefore, I went to a church and attended a healing service in which a "renowned healer" was to say prayers, give a lecture, and heal people. The flyers spoke of all the miraculous healings that had taken place because of this person. I wanted to go see him in action, pick up a few pointers, and maybe let him do his healing thing on me too.

The lecture was nice, the prayers genuine, and then came the clincher. Right before the actual healing service was to take place, the healer spoke of his books for sale, and many other articles that could be purchased in the back of the church. I began to feel mild amusement and skepticism.

When the usher came to my row for the healing part of the service, I marched down the aisle toward the front, along with the other people seeking miracles. I was instructed to stand with my arms down at my sides and there would be men behind me to "catch me in the Spirit" if I should fall from the Holy Spirit entering my body. I was ready, heart pounding, while the healer quickly moved toward me while he mumbled a few words of prayer (very few and said too low for me to hear) very rapidly over each person. Some of them fell backward and some just jiggled a bit. My turn came and went and I stood there, waiting for something miraculous to happen. I went ahead and fell backward to see if the men would catch me. They did and very gently, I was laid on the floor. The only thing I vividly recall is how cold the floor was, so I "raised up" as soon as I could and walked very "healed-looking" to the back of the church.

The tables full of religious articles awaited me in the back. The flurry of buying and selling was quite striking. Sales continued at a frenetic pace and the "healer" himself came back to the table and helped with the sales. The words "snake oil salesman" came into my mind. I shook my head sadly and slowly walked away. I do not judge him or question his motives or ability to heal, for that is God's job. I only know that my heart was saddened and I was disillusioned. Lord, was this what you wanted me to become? If so, I was going to say no thanks. I might as well go into acting. And I prayed.

April 8
I am gravely disturbed by what I witnessed by way of the so-called "healer" in church the other day in the name of God. I am so thoroughly disappointed. Is this how people heal others? I heard the Lord say to me, **"Heal for the sake of healing—my sake—not to become famous or wealthy. There are those who claim to heal but the flesh has taken over. Do not be like them. I provide what you need, including the why—when you are ready—patience."** From now on, I will be very careful in whom or to what I give my energy and belief.

April 24
I read something that addressed not worrying about the future. I asked the Lord about this and here was the reply. **"The future is NOW. All that happens is now and in the future—strung together like lights on a string. One light does not say, 'I am the now' and the light on the other end say, 'I am the future'. The entire string is lit up at one time. It is the present and the future, flowing together. Think and pray your future <u>now</u>. You cannot see it yet but the manifestation of it has begun. Keep believing. Do not stop the process. See it—feel it—the promise—my promise to you and yours. Continue to ask and believe. You will continue to give in ways you do not know and to receive in still other ways. Amen."** Oh, Lord, from your words, I see my future as healthy and whole—helping others as you direct me.

The Future is Now

The words of the Lord said it all. Do not keep waiting for something to begin to happen in the future. The future is already happening now. If I wanted to be healed, I had to believe that it had already begun, even if I didn't see it happening yet. For, if I were to believe it is somewhere "out there in the future," it would never occur. It would always be "in the future." The process is actually postponed or stopped by believing that it is not occurring right now. This was difficult for me. The statement, "Your future is now" always seemed like some sort of sales advertising slogan. I have realized that it is the truth. In the spiritual realm, there is no "time frame." I know that when we have a goal in mind, people will ask, "What is your time frame to get this accomplished?" I have to think differently to be healed. The "time frame" is now. God is already accomplishing the task. *Do not let this one fact escape your notice, beloved, that with the Lord one day is like a thousand years, and a thousand years like one day. (2 Peter 3:8)* God knows no time frame. Therefore, believe that what is needed and desired is already occurring right this minute. It is already being worked for a person if it is for the higher good. And how can being healed so that one can continue their life's role not be for the higher good? *For I know the plans that I have for you, declares the Lord, plans for welfare and not for calamity to give you a future and a hope. (Jeremiah 29:11)*

May 1

Today is 40 days after Easter—the day of the ascension of Jesus into heaven to return to the Father. It took awhile for the apostles to recognize him in his new glorified body. No wonder it takes us awhile to recognize His presence within each and every one of us.

I went to the clinic for a treatment today. I walked out the door and ran into Phil, director of the Living Beyond Disease ministry, associated with the clinic. We began chatting and he asked how I transitioned from being a retired school administrator to being in real estate. I laughed and explained how Lloyd had gotten into real estate and needed my help. I became a realtor to "help" him and ended up launching myself into a new career. I teasingly said, "I still don't know what I want to do when I grow up!" He chuckled and said, "Well, the first thing is not to grow up!" Then, he turned serious for a moment and said very thoughtfully, "Why don't your write your story?" I was dumbstruck. I have never been a writer. All I ever accomplished was helping one of my bosses write a scientific article, my Master's thesis, and then, later, my Doctoral dissertation, which were "just the facts, ma'am." I hastily replied, "Oh, sure. And why would anyone read it?" He answered, "You could give other people hope and we all love to read stories." I said, "Well, let me think about it." I was thinking there was no way in %&*% that I would write about something so very painful and personal for the world to see. He stated, "We could publish it for you." Now this was getting amazing. I remember that God said that all roads were being paved for me.

I am going to pray much on this. If it is of the Lord, I must do it. If it is my own ego responding, then the Lord must dispel it. O, Lord, I seek your help and counsel. Amen. *But if it is of God, you cannot overthrow it, lest you even be found to fight against God. (Acts 5:39)*

The Lord Paves the Way

Was this meant to be? I was flattered at the suggestion that I write down what had happened to me, but did I have the courage to share it with others? What if they made fun of me? What if I couldn't write anything other than scientific work? When I read St. Teresa of Avila's book, she revealed that she had been asked by her superiors to write about the "Interior Castle" of the soul.[1] She didn't want to do it, felt she would be ridiculed, and agonized much over it. She finally agreed, but still had to be cautious because of the "witch hunts" and the Inquisition going on during that period of time in history in Spain and around the world.

I, too, experienced some trepidation about such an undertaking. Selling real estate was much easier—sell a house and get paid or teach at the local university and get paid. If I entered completely new territory—write a book and what then? Have people think I was crazy because I heard the Lord? Would they think I was a religious fanatic? Or would they not believe that I was healed? Why would my story be any different than hundreds of other stories of recovery? So many questions entered my mind. Was this what the Lord meant when he said he had things planned for me?

The humorous part of me said, "Well, Diana, at least God didn't ask you to pack up your bags, sell all that you own, and move to Africa, Asia, or some other far away place to minister to the people. Also, you don't want to end up in the belly of a whale for saying no to God like Jonah in the Bible." God asked Jonah to go to Ninevah and tell the people to repent or they would be destroyed. He tried to avoid God's directive by hopping on a ship headed in some other direction. A storm came up, Jonah was thrown overboard, swallowed by a whale, and spent three days there in the dark before the whale spit him back out. He finally agreed to do God's bidding and went to Ninevah. The people repented and all was well.

I told myself, "You always tell other people not to be afraid when they ask the Lord to take over their lives. And look at YOU, you're afraid!" It became time to pray and to hope for some kind of answer. A marvelous coincidence was the presence of my journal. I tried unsuccessfully in the past to keep a journal. Why was I successful this time? Was this meant to be? Had God already been working the future in me by inspiring me to keep a journal of His words and my thoughts, feelings, and experiences? Was the fact that I kept a personal journal an example of "the future is now"? I was overwhelmed with amazement at how God works. He definitely puts in your heart what his plan is for you and you think that you thought of it yourself. In this case, it was revealed to me through His servant, Phil. The more I discovered, the more amazed I became. What do you think He is working in you and for you or your loved ones right at this moment? It's too awesome to know all at once. Watch the street of gold as it is paved before you.

May 2

I am still awestruck at what has been suggested to me by Phil—to write about my experiences. Is this a human effort or a Divine order? Jesus said, **"All humanity is both human and Divine. It is the humanity that is weak and the Divine that triumphs. This was my purpose—to show the triumph of my Father. All is never lost—only to those who wish it so. Do not see the world as it is—see My kingdom come. It is here but the hearts of man do not see it nor feel it. They are blinded by the darkness of their own hearts. Replace that darkness with my light and the kingdom appears. Pray—send out the light of my love as often as you can. There will always be a receiving heart. Remember, Divinity triumphs."**

It is now later in the day and I find myself still thinking and praying…mostly thinking. I sat down and tried to write one paragraph about my story from the beginning. The memory of the diagnosis and the horror of the chemotherapy were still so very painful. Thinking back on it gave me a horrible feeling in the pit of my stomach. No one should have to go through these things. I quit. I'm not meant to write. Lord, do you really want me to do this? The Lord answered me thus, **"I am laying it before you. Do not fear. All that I have said will come to pass. You will change hearts. That is the key. You will help people realize their love for me. This love has been blocked and you will help set it free. Live for me. I direct you. I am your healer and you are my healer—doing my work. You will know what to do soon. All is coming together. Trust me. I have saved the best for you. This is grace—my grace is what gives you confidence. Grace will not fail you. I will not fail you—believe and continue to claim my gifts. Amen."** *A highway will be there, a roadway, and it will be called the Highway of Holiness. The unclean will not travel on it. But, it will be for him who walks that way. And fools will not wander on it. (Isaiah 35:8)*

May 8
My abdomen is a little swollen right now and I've gained some weight. Fear is trying to overtake me because these were my symptoms before. The battle truly is in the mind. So, I prayed, "Oh, Jesus, sometimes I become afraid. I don't want to offend you by wavering in my belief of what you told me—that you would heal me. But, I am weak. Help me in my fear and weakness."

Jesus answered, **"I, your Lord, understand human weakness. I, too, suffered such weakness in the Garden of Gethsemane. Oh, to know what lay before me, knowing I had the power to change it, and yet knowing that it must take place for the good of all mankind. I, too, had to pray through the weakness. Pray—pray—pray until the calmness comes. That is what I did, even as my sweat turned into blood—the blood that would soon be shed for you and others. That is why, in my weakness, I asked my Father, that, if possible, this cup be removed from me.**

It was difficult being man, with all of the weaknesses, and the Son of God, *For all power was given to me in heaven and on earth, (Matthew 28:18)* **and yet, I had to surrender that power for the greater good. Oh, the agony this caused me. My father did not abandon me, nor does he abandon you. Stay steadfast in your faith. Pray through the darkness and the light appears. Amen"**

Setbacks May Happen

The revelation about the Garden of Gethsemane floored me. Jesus feeling fear and weakness—I forgot about that part of his life. I received renewed hope and understood that we are still human and consequently, have human weaknesses. I am usually a happy-go-lucky person. I never dwell on illness or fear, but this was no sprained ankle or bruised elbow. This was much more serious. I almost allowed this fear to be a setback to healing. In spite of what the Lord had promised me, what I "saw" with my eyes was attempting to frighten me out of my wits. I'd already been there and didn't want to go there again.

I went to the clinic for another treatment and talked to Melissa. "Look at this abdomen of mine! It is swollen and I am getting afraid."

"Diana, we have several patients who develop some bloating. When a person is undergoing any type of liver detoxification, there will be swelling as yeast, parasites, and other harmful bacteria die off."

"Are you sure?" (I had to ask my trademark question again—old habits are hard to break.)

"Yes. You are doing several things that detoxify the liver and swelling is something that can happen. Besides, you told me previously that the Lord has actually spoken to you and promised you healing."

"I know He has, but I still get scared at times."

"Hold on to what He told you. You heard Him speak. Hold on to that. You've got to."

"I am trying to, but sometimes I think it was just me talking to myself."

"It is not you talking to yourself. There is joy and peace and calm in what you hear. Trust what you have heard. Here's what we can do. You have two choices. You can have me take you off everything that detoxifies the liver and see your abdomen go down, or you can stay with the program and tough it out, despite what you see. What would you like to do?"

The choices hit me in the face. I think my friend from England calls it being "Gobsmacked." I was forced to make a decision—give in to the fear or press on—what would it be? I could hear her office clock relentlessly ticking in the silence as she waited patiently for my answer. I cannot begin to tell you the flood of thoughts going through my mind. I badly wanted physical proof that all was well, but I also needed to finish the regimen and be totally healed.

I sat with my head in my hands, confused again. Finally, I took a deep breath, after weighing the options, and said, "I am pressing through. Leave me on everything. I am going to trust the Lord and the process."

"Good for you, Diana. But, if you become the least bit afraid or concerned, call me, day or night."

"Do you really mean that—day or night? What if it's 3a.m. and I'm totally scared?"

"Call me. Patients do it all the time. I am able to fall back asleep." God reminded me that He, too, is available for listening day or night. I could do this.

May 11
The fear is trying to get me <u>again</u>— fears that I will not write down in this journal because I give them no power. Help me, Lord. **"Diana, you ARE healed."** Then, why, Lord, do I still have minor problems and setbacks? **"They are merely shudders and groans."** What do you mean by that? **"If a structure has been standing crooked for many years and it is renewed and placed upright slowly, the beams and timbers shudder and groan because they are reworked and made straight. So it is with you. It will be finished soon."** Thank you, Lord. I give my fears to you and accept the shudders and groans. Do not leave me. Let me continue to experience your presence. Amen. *When Peter saw how strong the wind was, he became frightened; and beginning to sink, he cried out, 'Lord, save me.' And immediately, Jesus stretched out his hand and caught him.(Matthew 14:30-3)* Catch me, Lord. Amen.

May 13
It has come to my attention lately, that after I hear the Lord's words, I either hear that same message from someone or I read it. So, what did I read today? In the book, The Cloud of Unknowing, I read these words, "A man...stands upright...so that

> he should figure forth in his physical appearance the spiritual work of the soul, which is spiritually upright and not crooked."[2] I get it! The shudders and groans are of the spirit! It is straining to come forth and be upright! Most enlightening!

A few weeks later, the swelling went down and my weight stabilized. I resolved that I would not give in to these fears that crept around me all of the time, looking for an entrance. I vowed to stay positive, expectant of good things, and patient for the results. I was ready for my spirit to be upright.

One of the books I read, *THE SECRET*, by Rhonda Byrne[3], stresses the importance of thinking about what you want and not focusing on what you don't want. She states that when you focus on what you don't like or don't want, more of it comes to you because you are giving your energy to that. Have you ever heard someone say, "I'm not going to waste my energy on that!"? Well, it's true! What you concentrate your energy on comes to fruition because your "energy" is a part of the "energy" of the Divine. Focus your energy on healing and what the new healthy you will look like. I drew a picture of my body with the long scar from surgery and everything else that was wrong with my body at that time. I got this idea from Melissa. Then, slowly, I began to use an eraser (it's best to draw it in pencil) and began to "erase" the things that needed to be gone and to draw in the things that needed to be there (like more hair on my head!). Now, I have a full head of hair and my long scar and other marks are hardly visible.

One of my lawyer acquaintances, Steve, used to ride a motorcycle. He said that bikers all know this rule. If you see a big pothole in the road ahead, do not focus on it. If you focus on it, you will aim right toward it and in you go. Therefore, as soon as you see the pothole, focus your eyes on the path around it and you will be safe. Great advice! I imagine it's the same concept with snow skiing and trees! Let's focus on the path around any "pothole" in life!

May 18
Today the Lord said to me, **"The work has begun. Start writing. The Holy Spirit guides you and the stories will fill in. You are a manifestation of me and I will be made manifest through your writing—begin. Begin to receive now all that I give you—no more delay. Be confident—let it flow. I direct all. Many souls need to hear. Sometimes, humans need other humans to 'connect with' until they are ready to 'connect' with me, to realize my presence. Think about how is has been for you—how something you heard or read by another human caused you to reflect and focus. So shall your words do to others. Amen."** I will do as you command, my Lord, with love, confidence, and humility. Give me the words. Amen

I wrote the first page and suffered through the near nausea of the all-too-recent memory. I feared that by writing my story and focusing on the first part, that I would set my body up for "re-entry" of malignant cells. The Holy Spirit remained there to help me through it. The results are what you are reading, after much inner searching and guidance from the Holy Spirit.

May 26
My mom and sister drove down from up north. It was so exciting to have them here and to spend time with my mom when neither one of us were in the hospital! She has recovered remarkably from her stroke and I love her so much. My sister Joann has been so supportive and we research the internet and other sources together since she is helping her husband, Myron, deal with his cancer. Lord, bless all of those who stand by and support their loved ones who are ill, even if it is with the smallest gesture of love.

We went to an Italian restaurant to celebrate mom's 79th birthday—hallelujah! To me, that celebration was more than just about my mom's birthday—it was a celebration of healing and life. It was a celebration of friendship and love. Thank you, Lord, for all of this. I know there are people who have lost their mothers or fathers and this is not possible for them. Touch their hearts also. Amen.

Supplements Fill Deficiencies

While eating at the restaurant for my mom's birthday, someone saw the extraordinarily large sized set of pills next to my plate and commented, "Are all of those pills part of your program?"

"Yes, they are."

"How many pills do you take in a day?"

"I take around 45-50 and some of them are harder to swallow. I am a person who never believed in taking supplements or pills of any kind and figured that my food would provide all that I needed. I also detest taking pills. So this was a huge change for me."

"And has this experience changed your mind?"

"Most definitely. Obviously, for me, some vital things were lacking, or I might not have developed this severe problem."

"Do you know what you were deficient in?"

"I do know that according to the books I've read, most people are deficient in one or more minerals. For many people, especially with serious diseases and conditions, it starts with a potassium deficiency. The body has a balance of sodium and potassium. Our diets are so heavily laden with sodium, that the body tries to flush it out and the potassium goes with it. So, the first thing the clinic did was to test my urine and saliva for potassium. They also had me eliminate as much salt from my diet as possible and take a potassium supplement. They monitor my potassium level in the urine. And for the amount of potassium that I need, eating bananas all day won't cut it."

"Interesting. What else do you take?"

"I take a calcium and magnesium pill four times a day. Many people don't get enough of those either. Calcium deficiencies are also linked to several health problems. And since dairy is forbidden on my eating plan, it becomes even more important. I also take selenium, Vitamin E, borage oil, and Omega 3 fish oil.

"Why don't you just eat lots of foods with these?"

"In my case, I am making up for what I didn't get in the past, plus trying to build my body up to get rid of anything that shouldn't be there. I'd have to eat fish every night to get all of the Omega 3 it takes to help the body overcome illness. Researchers have found that because people eat so many fried foods and the wrong fats, they are deficient in the good fats."

"Hard to believe there's such a thing as 'good' fats! What are those 3 smaller round ones and the other opaque pill?"

"Before I tell you that, let me say something. I have read in several articles and books that it is said, 'Death begins in the colon.' What you put in your mouth and how long it sits in your stomach and intestines both have a large impact on your health. It is imperative to have your food fully digested and to have healthy intestinal bacteria."

"And do any of those pills help with those things?"

"Two of the pills are full of digestive enzymes. Virtually all of us drink some liquid with our meal. This dilutes our own digestive enzymes and makes them work inefficiently. The food then sits in the stomach too long and begins to sour and ferment causing a myriad of problems like acid reflux, heartburn, nausea, and so forth. Just about everyone you know these days is on some type of prescription medicine for acid reflux or some other digestive tract problem. I take many supplements which have to be taken with food, so I do drink water with my meals. These enzymes really help get my food digested fully and reduce the acid reflux-like conditions. Certain digestive enzymes are responsible for breaking down the protective coating of cancer cells. The main enzymes that do this are typsin, chymotrypsin, and amylase. I also chew a few papaya tablets with chlorophyll just to make sure!"

"And the other pills?"

"One is a mixture of healthy bacteria such as lactobacillus and bifido bacteria. With all of the different foods we eat, we are taking in harmful bacteria all of the time. "Friendly bacteria" help keep the harmful bacteria from compromising the intestines. If the intestines are compromised, it can lead to ulcers and cancers. And the other pill is good old garlic. Here, smell it."

"Whew! That smells really strong! Remind me not to get in your face after you take that thing!"

"Supposedly, it doesn't give you bad breath, but definitely let me know if it does!" I said as I chuckled. Garlic has so many benefits that I can't tell you all of them in one sitting. But, to name a few, it helps lower cholesterol, actually kills tumor cells, and helps rebuild the liver."

"Aren't you glad we're Italians and we eat so much garlic? I might benefit from even more garlic in my food. Now, is everything I see here all that you take?"

"No, I also have some supplements that I take in tincture or liquid form. I take a liquid vegetable iron, and tincture of Echinacea, Red Root, Astragalus, and something called Scudder's Alterative. The Echinacea boosts the immune system, the Red Root helps clear out the lymph nodes, the Astragalus helps boost immune capacity and inhibit the metastasis of cancer cells, and the Scudder's Alterative helps change the body tissues to make them less friendly to harmful substances. I take 40 drops of Milk Thistle to detoxify my liver. But, I can tell you, when mixed all together, they taste AWFUL. So, I put all of them in my fake coffee and drink it down."

"It must be tough swallowing all of those pills and taking liquids that taste bad."

"You know, it IS tough. But, the alternative to taking all of these is either chemotherapy or remaining in a state of unbalance or illness and in my case, I felt that it was absolutely necessary to my healing. May I tell you a quick story?"

"Sure!"

"I watched a program on the Discovery® Channel on television about how they make white bread. They take the current wheat grain, which has 3 parts and remove all of the wheat germ (inner part) and the bran (outer layer). These are the two healthiest parts. They sell the wheat germ to health food stores. Then, they grind up what is left, the endosperm. Endosperm is the middle layer full of carbohydrates, which is treated to make it white. Finally, they ADD iron, niacin, and a few other ingredients back into it.

The information that they left out, I read in a nutritional book. After they remove the wheat germ and bran, what do you think is left? Nothing nutritional! It has absolutely no nutritional value at this point. Companies would not be able to sell bread as a food item if they did not add something back into it! After they artificially add ingredients, it is now a "processed food." We eat lots of foods like that. It's no wonder to me that we get deficient in nutrients and need to take supplements. And, the fact that they sell the wheat germ and bran to health food stores ought to tell us all something!"

"I knew there was a reason that I don't eat white bread any more, but I wasn't really sure what it was until you just explained it."

"And guess what else?"

"What?"

"Foods like that have very little to no fiber. They "clog up" the intestines. Food sits in there and moves along the digestive tract VERY slowly. It was fun when we were kids and we would take pieces of bread and roll them into "dough balls"! That's about what processed bread does in the intestines—gums up and balls up. The longer food sits in the intestines, the more harmful substances (like pesticides, preservative chemicals, etc.) get absorbed into the cells, and some foods (like meats) actually begin to rot and ferment. You can imagine how the disease process is beginning from all of this. In the average person, it may take 3 or 4 days for food to get from one end to the other."

"Is that why all of the television commercials now show how much fiber they are adding to different foods?"

"I imagine that is the case. But, it makes an even better case to eat lots of whole foods in the form of fruits and vegetables with fiber—just one of the reasons why I eat at least one-half to one apple a day, for example. Whole foods mean those foods that are completely in their natural state. I read a book called, *You Can Heal Your Life* by Louise Hay[4]. She says that if it doesn't grow, she doesn't eat it."

"And yet another item I take is called Neprinol®. It helps destroy fibrin. Fibrin can be found in scar tissue or other places where bleeding has occurred. Fibrin is manufactured in the liver and if the liver isn't working properly, too much can be produced, clogging arteries, etc. Neprinol also contains serra-peptase, which helps destroy the outer stealth coating of cancer cells. The stealth coating is what cancer cells develop to outsmart the immune system into not destroying them as a foreign body. Finally, I take inositol and IP6."

"Hey, thanks for all of the information. Would you help me with some resources on supplements some time?

"Sure—I'd be honored. I could tell you so much, it would make your head spin. It makes MY head spin at times! But, enough of that, it looks like it's time to sing Happy Birthday to mom! Tanti auguri a te, tanti auguri a te...." (Happy Birthday to you in Italian)

According to Patrick Quillin, PhD[5], more than 40% of cancer patients actually die from malnutrition, most Americans are deficient in vitamins, and there is a widespread deficiency of minerals. Part of it is due to the depletion of our soils in many essential minerals. We now add chemicals to our soil as fertilizer instead of the natural fertilizers (such as cow manure) that farmers once used. We eat fast foods and not enough of the fresh food.

Quillin states that if you have a headache, you are not deficient in aspirin. If you have cancer, you are not deficient in chemotherapy or radiation, but you are deficient in SOMETHING. Sometimes these deficiencies produce early warning signs such as a craving for something like pickles or a strange non-food craving such as eating chalk or talcum powder. A body with no deficiencies has no disease and no 'cravings'. A sugar craving can also be a sign of too much yeast, cancer, or other ill condition in the body. I encourage you to do your own research, talk with your local health food providers about your needs, and do what is necessary to fully provide for the needs of your cells. You will marvel at the renewed results and energy.

Heavenly Pearls of Wisdom

Pray for courage. The courage to allow yourself to be healed and the courage to help others heal.

The future is now. Expect the healing process to be occurring in you at this very moment.

God paves the way. It happens effortlessly. What you need unfolds before you...let it unfold.

Setbacks may happen. Pray through them and stay with the healing program the Lord has led you to.

Nutritional supplements are a good thing. We eat tons of processed food, devoid of nutrition. We must make it up somehow.

Check out any cravings. They are not a good sign. Something is amiss. Catch it now.

8
The Manifestation of God

June 4
A friend of mine, Kim, is scheduled for surgery on Friday to remove a non-malignant brain tumor. It started with a disturbance in her hearing. What is happening to all of us? I will sit in the waiting room and pray. I pray, O Lord, that your hand will extend over all and that you guide all of those working on Kim to success and complete recovery for her.

June 7
Kim had surgery yesterday. She came through the surgery well, but today she is unable to swallow or speak. The tumor had been wrapped around the nerves that control these sensations also. She has a long slow recovery ahead of her and doctors are unsure of whether she will get all of her hearing back. Lord, be with her and her husband and see them through this tough time.

Artificial Sweeteners

I feel the need at this point, and considering what has happened with Kim, to address artificial sweeteners, since they seem to be related to tumors of the brain. They come under various names, but I am only going to mention three or four of them here. Every bit of research that I have seen either pronounces these as downright dangerous or at best, long term effects are still being investigated. Quillin, in *BEATING CANCER WITH NUTRITION*[1], reports that Aspartame, marketed as Equal™ or NutraSweet™, has been linked to a 250% rise in brain cancer since its approval in 1981. Saccharin increases bladder cancer in animal studies, and Acesulfame K, sold as Sunette™ or Sweet One™, reveals cancer problems in early studies. Splenda™ was approved in 1998, but there are currently not enough published long-term studies available to make a judgment.

I am not saying that my friend had a brain tumor because of artificial sweeteners, but I am saying we KNOW that certain ones are dangerous. Avoid them! Lloyd and I use very little sugar and try to avoid lots of sweets, desserts, and so on. But, if we do want a little sweetness in our Japanese green tea, which we drink iced, we add Agave syrup, available in most stores. It is similar to honey, but will dissolve in cold liquids. Give up those diet drinks!

One of the goals in overcoming any "disease", or to keep from developing a problem, is to maintain a constant blood sugar level. Spikes in blood sugar set the stage for all sorts of problems. It is most desirable to achieve a level of "homeostasis", which means keeping the body within a certain range for blood sugar, acid-base balance, temperature, and so forth.

June 27

Today I prayed and the Lord answered me as he always does. Oh, Father, I feel so conflicted. There is so much I want to give, so much I want to DO, so many worthy causes to which I wish I had more money to give. He said, **"All in good time, Diana. I shower blessings upon you. Blessings come in many forms and ways. You shall see."** Lord, you have already blessed me in so many ways beyond my dreams. **"And yet more is yours for the asking. I am the endless supply. If only people would trust me for their supply. I can provide**

all things. Nothing good is accomplished without me. I am all." I believe, Lord. I thank you for your encouragement. I wish so badly to heal others. **"I encourage you because I love you. You are still learning to trust what you cannot see."** *Praise be to the God and Father of our Lord Jesus Christ, the father of compassion and the God of all comfort, who comforts us in all our troubles, so that we can comfort those in any trouble with the comfort we ourselves have received from God. (1 Corinthians 1: 3-4)* I repent, Lord, of not believing. I repent of all 'nots'. **"You are always forgiven. Now, go forth and reveal my glory. Amen."**

My friend Pam who delivers my Avon came by and she is totally finished with chemotherapy and radiation. She says she still doesn't feel up to par yet, but has been pronounced free and clear of the cancer. Now she will continue to go for check-ups. I am glad that this worked out for her, as she has been through a lot after being hospitalized with the infection and receiving blood. Now she and her husband plan to resume their traveling.

June 30

Today is Andraya's 30th birthday. Thank you, Lord, for giving me renewed life and the ability to share earth's milestones with my loved ones. You are awesome, as we say in today's lingo. But, Lord, today, I come to you because I want to know what grace is and to "feel" it. I pray for wisdom to share with others. How do I know if I am letting grace flow? I'm beginning to wonder what grace is. How do we know if and when we have any?

"My grace is upon you. Let my grace lead all that you are and all that you do." Lord, I hope that I am doing just that. But, I think I need grace lessons. **"They come every day—be alert. Grace is what turns a bad situation into something good. Grace heals a heart that is broken, sad, depressed,**

> **angry, or hopeless. Grace lets the words flow to soothe others. Grace changes non-believers into believers. What you call a miracle is simply a flow of grace. It is not tangible or visible. It just IS. It is like water flowing. It is of me. Grace allows you to be the Christ-like being that I created. Grace lifts the veil over your eyes so that you begin to see in the spirit. Let that Grace lead you today and every day. Amen."**
> *May our Lord Jesus Christ himself and God our father who loved us and by his grace gave us eternal encouragement and good hope... (2 Corinthians 2:16)*

Recognizing Grace in our Lives

When God said that His grace was upon me, I wondered why I didn't "feel" any different. I expected to be walking on clouds, have a halo over my head, or to see something visible at least. The Bible states, *From the fullness of his grace we have all received one blessing after another. (John 1:16).* Grace—we all have received it. If the future is indeed now, grace is already working in you and me at this moment. We may not "feel" it with our senses, but it IS there. We take grace in and we pass it on. I never thought that an encouraging word I say to someone is an example of grace flowing. That is God working through us. When we give someone a heartfelt hug, that is grace. My search is over. I know that grace is everywhere and in me. It's such a natural part of what is given to us that we don't think about it or "feel" it as something different. If we stop the flow, then God's grace dies within us. It must flow out from us, even if it is just in thought. All we have to do is think a pleasant thought and wish another well and that, too, is an invisible flow of grace.

Because of the presence of the Divine in us, we are constantly bringing about miracles. Some miracles are small, some are big, and some occur much later in earth time. *So, Paul and Barnabas spent considerable time, speaking boldly for the Lord, who confirmed the message of his grace by enabling them to do miraculous signs and wonders.*

(Acts 14:3) The Lord revealed to me that grace helps people believe. To me, that means that every time I have an "Aha!" moment of learning some truth or believing something, it is God's grace that performed that feat. *On arriving, he (Apollos) was a great help to those who by grace had believed. (Acts 18:27)* Therefore, we know that God's grace is constantly working in us and that the process is to be trusted. It flows through us in the way we are—our character. It also flows in how we treat others and how we deal with situations.

The more sickness and sin increase, the more God sends us his grace. He never sends us a sickness, but if we get what appears as one, he sends us the grace we need to become enlightened. He sends us the grace to pray for help, then he sends us grace in the form of help, watches the grace unfold in us, and then watches us pass that grace on to others. *The law was added so that the trespass might increase. But where sin increased, grace increased all the more... (Romans 5:20)*

It is grace that gives you the talents you have and grace that will help you uncover even more talents. *We have different gifts, according to the grace given us. (Romans 12:6)* You and I each have a unique gift and using that gift allows more grace to flow. Illness and the recovery process made me more thankful for each and every gift and talent. A talent might be something as simple as being able to organize, cook, keep a house clean, work with children, and so on. They are all talents. Our society sometimes downplays the value of certain talents, but they are all talents given by God, nevertheless.

And last, even though the incidences of grace are boundless, is the use of grace to heal. You and I have all the grace we need to be healed as long as the grace isn't blocked. If we are still having little family squabbles, or still resenting someone, grace is blocked. Practicing forgiveness and repentance every day becomes part of the healing process. *And the God of all grace, who calls you to his eternal glory in Christ, after you have suffered a little while, will himself restore you and make you strong, firm and steadfast. (I Peter 5:10).*

July 6
I had read a passage in the Bible. It said that the Jewish people had implored God because Heliodorus was going to attack their treasury. But, just as he approached, *...the Lord of spirits who holds all power manifested himself in so striking a way that those bold enough to follow Heliodorus were panic stricken. There appeared to them a richly caparisoned horse, mounted by a dreadful rider...wearing golden armor. (2 Maccabees 3:24)*

So, I told the Lord, "Wow, it would be so awesome to see you manifested in some neat way like that." He answered me with this, **"I am manifested in everything you see, even the little birds that come to your bird feeders every day—they are all manifestations of me."** I was in awe that I had been reminded that these creatures, ALL living creatures, and all beauty were manifestations of God. Today, I was watching the birds at my birdfeeder and the most beautiful bird appeared with a blue head, green back, red throat, and bright orange belly. Never in the 9 years that we've lived here have I seen this beautiful bird. I found out it is called a painted bunting. I knew that God sent this bird to reaffirm his striking manifestation. May all of us be a striking manifestation of you, O God. Thank you for what you showed me today.

How God Manifests

A part of me wanted proof of God's presence and beauty. When the spirit hurts or is weak, its desire to know and experience God becomes very strong. As spiritual beings, we perceive our relationship with the Creator. However, the fleshly portion of us wants "proof." The message God gave pointed out the fact that what we seek, is, in fact, figuratively in our own back yard.

God shows himself in all the beauty around us. Every time we see a bird, butterfly, or the smallest insect, that is God being made manifest. When we hear a donkey bray (the neighbor behind us owns one), an owl hoot, or a bird sing, think of our Lord. In O'Donnell's book *OF MONKEYS AND DRAGONS, FREEDOM FROM THE TYRANNY OF DISEASE*[2], she encourages us to be a beholder. If we concentrate on beholding what God shows us, it awakens us and heals our spirit. In the Bible, Matthew quotes what the prophet said, *Behold, the virgin shall be with child and bear a son, and they shall call his name Emmanuel, which means 'God with us.' (Matthew 1:23)* We notice that the prophet speaks of beholding or being astonished at this news. He doesn't say listen or look, but behold. The word "behold" is mentioned several times.

I asked the Lord many years ago to reveal to me the closest visible item resembling heaven that we experience on earth. I waited patiently, did not receive an immediate answer, and forgot all about it. Several weeks later, I was driving down the highway to another city just after it had rained and "beheld" the most beautiful rainbow. Instantly, I knew in my being that this was God's answer to my question. And I said, "Thank you, God. It is absolutely beautiful! What heaven must be like—none of us can imagine." A rainbow is but a faint shadow of God's beauty and look how breath taking it is. *Behold the rainbow! Then bless its Maker, for majestic indeed is its splendor. It spans the heavens with its glory this bow bent by the mighty hand of God. (Sirach 43:10-12)*

After receiving that astonishing answer, I boldly asked God what the most heavenly sound is that we have on earth. I was very surprised by the answer. It was not the sound of trumpets blaring, nor the sound of harps playing, as we often hear in the movies. It was not any musical instrument. It was the sound of children's voices singing, especially singing praises to the Lord. That might explain why choirs of children are so enthralling to many. When we hear a child's voice, it represents innocence and purity which are beautiful parts of God. *At that time the disciples came to Jesus and said, "Who then is greatest in the kingdom of heaven?" And he called a child to himself and set him before them, and said, Truly I say to you, unless you are converted and become like children, you will not enter the kingdom of Heaven. Whoever humbles himself, then, as this child, he is the greatest in the kingdom of Heaven. (Matthew 18: 1-4)*

How does God manifesting Himself help me to heal? Taking moments to "behold" the simplest of God's creations fills us with awe and wonder. When we are beholding in this ethereal state, we are finding the peace within our soul that allows healing to occur. It also takes our mind off of our own condition or problems and that alone is refreshing.

View yourself, also, as a manifestation of God—because you are. All that is your "essence" is God manifesting Himself through and as you. As a manifestation of Him, you are meant to be whole and perfect. You deserve to be nothing less. Your job is to accept this gratefully as God's gift.

Become aware and develop an awe of all that is around you and within you. As O'Donnell says, we must behold the goodness of God, that everything we see in nature is there for us, and that God continues to reveal Himself to us about our true existence[3].

August 1

I went to the clinic and talked to Melissa about leg cramps. If only I had appreciated the days when I was younger and, at times, absolutely nothing was wrong with my body and nothing hurt. Too bad wisdom has to come with age. I hope I can return my body to those types of days. Why can't we appreciate all that we have at an earlier age? Well, anyway, Melissa said it is time for some more blood work. So, I asked if I should go ahead and get a CA-125 test, the cancer marker. The last one I had was in May over a year ago. She turned the question over to me and asked me if I was ready. I didn't know what to say. I became afraid and confused. Should I have the test? Was I confident enough in what God had told me? If

I didn't like the results, would I panic? So, I told her that I didn't want the test yet. I think the reason that I feel pressured to be tested is because all of my friends and relatives keep asking if I have any tests as proof that I am healed yet. We all want proof of the manifestation.

This morning I prayed and as I read in my Bible about the ascension of Jesus into heaven on a cloud, these words came to my heart, **"It is time for your resurrection. It is time for your proof. The proof of my glory made manifest through you and others like you so that all may believe even though they have not seen. Continue to give glory to my name.**

I am a God of mercy and compassion—not just one of thunder and lightning, but a God of WHISPERS and ROSES. Accept this rose of love and health from one who loves you. People do not give me credit for all that I am. You must be my spokesperson. Do as I command. I send the Holy Spirit upon you just as I did for the apostles on Pentecost. Preach far and wide to anyone who will listen. I am behind and before you. Go forth with confidence. Amen." Lord, I thank you and love you very much. I am so grateful for all that you have done for me and all that you are. *A strong wind was rending the mountains and crushing rocks before the Lord, but the Lord was not in the wind. After the wind was an earthquake, but the Lord was not in the earthquake. After the earthquake, there was fire, but the Lord was not in the fire. After the fire there was a tiny whispering sound. When he heard this, Elijah hid his face in his cloak. (I Kings 19:11-13)*

I just know that I am going to either receive a rose or see a rose as a result of God's words to me. Time will tell. I felt the very tender sweet love of God, just as if he had assumed human form, knelt in front of me, and presented me with a rose of love. It was so awesome. I don't think we realize the tenderness and sweetness of the Lord. He is certainly correct when he says that we don't give him the credit for all that he is.

August 10

I have been getting therapeutic body massages since I read that they are an important part of healing. They release toxins and help the body to revive. While I was in the massage room, I noticed that the massage therapist had a statue of an angel on the desk. Next to the statue of the angel was a vase with a single rose in it. But it was not an ordinary rose, it was made of chocolate and wrapped in red foil. Knowingness hit me immediately. I knew that this was a sign from the Lord of his offer to me of a rose of health and love, when he said "Whispers and Roses." What a wonder God is! He knows my fondness for chocolate and for flowers. The Lord always provides encouragement in many forms just when I need it. I will ask him to make me aware. I accept the rose of health and healing, Lord. *And he who loves me will be loved by my father, and I will love him and manifest myself to him. (John 14:21)*

August 13

I received a devastating e-mail today. My friend and Avon lady, Pam, passed away from cancer. O, Lord. How can this be? She had chemotherapy and radiation and had been pronounced free and clear. What happened? I cry out to you once again. Let the truth be known, spread, and accepted of who we are and what you have placed upon this earth to cure those in need. Have mercy on us.

I want to see my friends live. Answer our plea—end the needless suffering. What are the drug companies, food manufacturers, and the medical community doing to us? Is it for healing or for money and profit? If it is for profit, woe to them, Lord, woe to them. Are they so willing to instill fear in us by imposing a treatment that is worse than death and seems to hasten it? My very spirit weeps and is broken. I have lost another friend. I love you, Pam. You are now perfect and whole in Him and may you share in His glory. Amen.

August 16
I attended the memorial service for Pam and was able to speak with her husband. I asked him what had happened when just two months earlier she had been pronounced free and clear of cancer. He stated that she had begun to complain of back pain and went to the doctor in July. After some tests, the doctor informed her that the cancer had returned and was on her spine, liver, and several other places—that she was terminal. Terminal! They had given her a 70% chance of survival—it shows me that they don't know anything. People put 100% of their trust in them and they know nothing! They merely make a stab at a dartboard with these percentages of survival.

The doctors gave her two choices—either to do nothing and have Hospice care or try more chemotherapy and hope for the best. She chose chemotherapy. The first dose knocked her for a loop. The second dose landed her in the hospital and she never recovered. Her husband said the chemotherapy killed her. I wanted to tell him that they had a third choice which was to call me or the holistic clinic I attended, but she knew the treatment I had chosen because we had talked of it many times when she delivered my Avon supplies. Another cinnamon roll boiled in the oil while I stood helplessly by, unable to help. My heart is heavy—so heavy—fill us with your truth, Lord. Amen.

Surrounded by the Enemy

This was now twice that I had lost a friend in the past few months. I sent monthly electronic mail updates to all of my friends and relatives. I talked to anyone who would listen about the holistic approach. I read every book put before me about nutritional foods, alternative therapies, and spiritual help. I am still reading books. I am still learning. I am still growing spiritually. But, I realize that I cannot interfere with the choices that my friends and relatives make, even when I see that it causes their bodily demise. It is not our fault. While enjoying the quiet the other morning, it came to me that by noon, most of us have taken in or been exposed to hundreds of chemicals. We didn't have these long ago! They have crept into our lives ever so slowly.

Let me do a quick mental list. I will probably miss something that you will think of as you read this. First thing in the morning, folks wash their face or take a shower. There are chemicals in the water ranging from metals to chlorine to pesticide runoff. The new PVC (polyvinylchloride) pipes give off gases. The soap we use is full of chemicals (if in doubt, read the label.) The shampoo and conditioner are chemicals and the shaving cream is a pile of chemicals. Body lotions contain chemicals, toothpaste contains chemical compounds, make up contains chemical concoctions such as parabens and phthalates, hairspray and hair gel are chemicals. Deodorant usually contains aluminum and other chemicals. That last morning spritz of perfume or cologne adds another layer of chemicals. The skin is a major organ that absorbs much more than we ever think about, sending these chemicals into the blood stream and eventually to every cell in our body.

The morning cup of java and fresh fruit contain pesticides, the breakfast cereal has chemical additives, pesticide residues, and so do many processed foods. If you cooked your food in a coated pan, Teflon™ escapes from the scratches into the food. The digestive system is another place where nutrients and other items that aren't nutrients are absorbed and carried to the liver and cells. The soap to wash the dishes contains even more chemicals which leave some residue. Next, we head to work in the traffic and gas fumes that we breathe in. The lungs are yet another absorption point.

Lloyd and I traveled to Italy to see my relatives and go sightseeing. We have seen the famous canals of Venice and eaten at the restaurants, including one of the "American" fast food restaurants located not too far from St. Mark's Square. A book about the burning of an opera house in Venice, Italy, by John Berendt, called *The City of Fallen Angels,* contains a story about one of the city's famous rat pest control experts. Rats would forage in the garbage behind the city's restaurants and became quite a nuisance because they were multiplying like crazy. The "Rat Man of Treviso," by the name of Massimo Donadon, would set out his usual traps filled with the rats' favorite Italian food laced with rat poison. He fed American rats a diet of vanilla, granola, popcorn, and margarine. He had observed that "Rats eat what people eat."[4]

He noticed something different about the eating habits of the Italian rats. Fast food restaurants (which have invaded all of Europe) had taken hold in Italy. "I've noticed," he said, "that in the past few years Italian rats have begun to prefer eating plastic to Parmesan cheese...Plastic is the rats' equivalent of fast food!"[5] Apparently, they could not distinguish between fast food, which Massimo called non-food, and plastic. Eureka! He promptly bought some shredded plastic, laced it with the poison coumarin, killed many rats, and had a booming business. He was also very pleased that it was much cheaper to feed the rats plastic than Parmesan cheese! What does this say to us? I first read this as simply an amusing story of Venice, but now I am beginning to fully realize the significance of the situation and how it relates to us.

If rats confuse food with plastic, the nutritional value of certain fast foods must be severely lacking. You may be thinking, "Yeah, but rats will eat anything!" Rats actually have very similar nutritional requirements to humans and that is why they are often selected as "participants" in various laboratory studies of drugs, nutrients, and other items humans consume. Don't we all know many humans who will also eat anything? The chemical composition of fast food would be a most interesting study. We always joke about the discovery of margarine and its original intended non-food function and now we have embraced it as "food". It is claimed that it is one molecule away from being plastic. Coincidence? Makes me shudder. I am staying with butter and just using it sparingly, or better yet, olive oil.

We have problems with the plastic Melamine. It was reported recently that it was found in baby formula! The FDA has not condemned this because they have not established harmful levels of the plastic yet. How can ANY amount of plastic be tolerable or even acceptable for an infant? Melamine in cat food has already killed many cats. The FDA is supposed to protect us! *You have seen many things, but have paid no attention; your ears are open, but you hear nothing. (Isaiah 42:20)*

Is it any wonder that we are seeing more and more diseases? The liver becomes overloaded with the chemicals and impurities it removes from the blood stream. Once the liver becomes overwhelmed, it is no longer able to remove the impurities from the blood and they are then allowed to enter the cells of the body and to interfere with vital cell and life functions. The blood then becomes "impure." And what does the medical community encourage? They prescribe more chemicals for a body that is already overloaded to the point of disease. I often wondered why certain drugs say that one must check the liver periodically. The manufacturers KNOW that the drugs cause liver damage! Something is wrong here.

When I first became a real estate agent, I thought about the fact that I would be going over contracts and offers with clients. I wanted my nails to look really spiffy so I went to the local nail salon and had a manicure. But, with the way I constantly have my hands in water or reaching in my purse for things, the nail polish wore off and looked ragged too quickly. I went back to the nail salon and had them put on those acrylic nails with nail polish (more chemicals). They were so beautiful and I couldn't help but admire them. The only problem is that after about two "fills", the nails have to be removed and new ones put on. I shudder to think back about how they would give me a bowl of acetone and have me soak my fingers in there for about 20 minutes! Think of all of the chemicals being absorbed into my skin! Acetone causes skin problems, headaches, and other problems. I am no longer getting my nails done and due to the supplements, my nails are no longer brittle, but nice and strong.

What can we do? We can begin to make different choices. If you have the presentation of an illness, you must begin to make changes. There are filters for the water, even for bath water and showers. One can drink chlorine-free or other filtered water. There are natural soaps, make-up, lotions, hair products, deodorant, cleaners, and toothpastes available. One can also find at least some organic vegetables in the supermarket. It's still a small expensive section, but there is always hope. It is a costly, lengthy process for a company to be given the "certified organic" label and that is why the price is so high. You might even grow a few of your own vegetables or fruits.

There are herbs that have profound healing benefits with no side effects. I was surprised to find a good herbalist near me. The local health food store contains jars of herbs and usually, one can find a knowledgeable store employee to help. There are even herbal hair dyes. I don't get my nails done anymore. I'd rather have plain nails or once in awhile, a little polish.

Once we make these and other changes, we cannot force our friends and relatives to do the same and get on board. We can give them information, direct them to resources, and pray for them. That is all God asks of us. Each person comes to the truth in different ways and at different times as the story of their life unfolds. If they ask you for information or help, that is another matter. You have been given an opening and an opportunity and are obligated by the Lord to assist them. This happened to me on many occasions.

On other occasions, people heard what I was doing, asked no questions, and showed no interest. I let them be. If you are reading this, then you are already beginning to change and awaken. May you continue forward on your path of holiness.

Heavenly Pearls of Wisdom

Give up the artificial sweeteners. God never intended for such chemicals to be ingested. That is why he gave us honey and agave nectar.

Grace is all around you. Ask God to help you become more aware, especially for healing. He loves sending it to you—as much as you need.

Take note of God's manifestation. It is for you to behold and to help you heal. Be in awe of every thing.

Reduce your exposure to chemicals. Begin with one or two items at a time and switch to organic vegetables and products as it becomes possible.

Do not try to convert others. The harder you try, the more they will rebel. If they ask for help, do all you can.

9
Channel of God's Grace

August 18

I had a dream last night that I was dressed and ready to go somewhere, but I discovered that I had no shoes on my feet. I didn't know what to do and was very distraught. Someone (I don't remember who) gave me a beautiful pair of bright pink sandals to wear. They were absolutely beautiful. I noticed that they didn't match my dress, but I didn't care. They were so striking. At our Monday night meeting at the clinic, Rosella (an attendee of the meetings) talked about how it says in the Bible that when the prodigal son returned, he was given a ring of authority, a robe, and a new pair of sandals. Most interesting! I later told Michele O'Donnell about my dream and she said that it's time to start walking the path and doing what the Lord has set out for me to do. Most fascinating!

Dear Lord, I am yours. I am ready to do your will—to help others—but do they really want to be helped? **"The ones that desire help will be sent to you."** Work through me, Lord, to heal them and renew my spirit. **"It is already done."**

Your Story Walks God's Path

But the father said to the servants, "Bring out the best robe and put it on him, and put a ring on his hand, and sandals on his feet." (Luke: 15:22)

I can certainly identify with the prodigal son who became impatient and demanded that his father give him his share of his inheritance now. He promptly went out, traveled around, and spent it all. He came begging back to the father who welcomed him back with open arms and even had a big feast in his honor. I, too, had been "gone" for a period of my life, and returned.

Many years ago, in trying for our second child, I lost a set of twins who were born too early. One was born dead and the other died of hyaline membrane disease, despite the doctor's efforts to save him. I didn't even get to hold him or see him before he died. Never in my life up to this point had anyone close to me passed away. And now, just a few days after giving birth, I was faced with choosing a casket and planning a funeral. I didn't understand why this had happened to me. Sadness was a part of my daily life from that moment forward, but I still had hope in life and the Lord. The doctors assured me that this was a once in a blue moon type of event.

I became pregnant again two years later and the doctor was extra vigilant. All exams went well, all appeared normal, and delivery day came. The baby boy was delivered and an hour later, the doctor returned with a somber face and tears in his eyes to tell me that little Anthony (the name I had given him) had a severe heart problem and would require immediate surgery to try and save his life. The nurses brought him by my bed in his incubator, all hooked up to tubes and oxygen, and I sobbed to see him struggling to breathe. The doctors performed surgery but Anthony died the next day. Once again, I'd never gotten the chance to hold my baby. And again, we had to select a casket, bury him next to his brother, and select a headstone. This wasn't how life was supposed to be. Not in the books I'd read.

I was devastated emotionally, physically, and spiritually. I was angry with God—very angry. I was so angry that I turned my back on Him, believed he was punishing me for something I hadn't done, and refused to give Him any praise and glory. One bad experience I could understand, but not two. That was unforgivable. The "kind" words of others such as, "Don't worry, you'll have another child," or "It's good that Anthony passed before you got to know him," only renewed my grief.

I attended church services for awhile to keep up appearances but my heart wasn't in it. My heart ached and the sadness overwhelmed me. I blamed God for everything wrong in my life. I stopped going to church. But, for some reason, before I went to bed on many nights I said, "God, I'm still angry with you but please don't give up on me." Even when I had a baby girl two years later (Andraya), I still didn't trust Him. I rebelled, didn't pray much, and spiritually remained "disconnected".

God didn't give up on me. He kept gently nudging me and finally, I began to go to church again. I went on a spiritual retreat several years later and became renewed. God had welcomed me back like the prodigal son. When I received the cancer diagnosis several years later, I didn't blame God. I didn't say "why me?" I didn't become angry and I didn't turn my back on Him. In fact, I turned toward Him and His mercy because I know that turning away from God is never the answer. My relationship with God had changed and continues to change. For me, God went from being the God of the Old Testament who was <u>outside</u> of me to the God of the New Testament who was <u>inside</u> of me and worked through me. God hasn't changed. I am the one changing. I know that he didn't send something like that to me. He is all goodness and he NEVER changes.

Where does that leave us? For me, it means putting on the new sandals. It means walking on the path as it unfolds. God uses our story for his greater good and glory. Every one of our lives is a story. Even small acts can be for the glory of God, as St. Paul tells us: *Whether, then, you eat or drink, or whatever you do, do all to the glory of God.(I Corinthians 10:31)* We jokingly say that our lives are a "soap opera", but I would rather think of my life as God's adventure. Whatever adversity we face in our life, the challenge is to stay on GOD'S PATH. If we wander off of the path and refuse the help of the Lord, we are headed for nothing but trouble and heartache. I've already been there and I choose life, belief in the Lord, and hope. Stay the course.

August 22

It is good to repent every night before I go to bed, blessing everyone. I sleep with a clear conscience. O, Lord, I repent of anything that I have done today or lately that is displeasing to you. And I thank you for all you have done for me. **"Diana, you have healed away the years. You are a new creation—remember that. Once the truth is made known, people will experience a change. Some do not wish to change because they have become comfortable with the veil of untruth over their eyes, so they choose to ignore what is right in front of them. Do not despair, little one. All that you do is of great consequence in the kingdom. I chose you and you answered me. That is pleasing to me. I call many who do not answer and do not obey."** I am here, Lord, to serve you only. You alone are my savior. Amen. *You did not choose me, but I chose you and appointed you to bear fruit and that your fruit should remain, that whatever you ask the Father in my name, He may give you. (John 15:16)*

God Has Chosen You

It is hard for us ordinary people to believe that God actually "chooses" us. God chooses each one of us to carry out his will, be a light to others, pray, and use the graces He gives us as talents to serve others. However, he also has chosen you to grow in the spirit. You have been seeking and now you have been chosen, as partly evidenced by the fact that you are reading this.

You have been called out of your personal desert, your period of wandering, your exile in Egypt. According to Thomas Merton, a Trappist monk who wrote *THE SEVEN STOREY MOUNTAIN*, once you have been called out of your Egypt, you cannot live as you lived there. Your former life and self have been crucified.[1] It is now time to head toward the promised land—your spiritual awakening. You are like a young chick pecking furiously to get out of its "shell". God helps you out and once you are free, He expects great things from you. You are up to the task and you have been chosen.

You may ask, "What have I been chosen to do or be?" That, my friend, you must seek as an answer from the Lord. I remember going through all of the ministries in the church bulletin trying to find what the Lord wanted me to "do". What a frustrating endeavor it was for me! There were several choices and I read each one carefully, pondering, praying. I could go visit the prisoners, write letters to the prisoners, serve soup to the homeless, make hope chests, sew blankets for babies, make care packages for the troops, collect clothing for the needy, lead a Bible study group, teach religion to the youngsters, go to the nursing home for services, sew pillows for teenage mothers, or join a prayer group.

I "tried out" a couple of these ministries and nothing "clicked". When it is God's calling for you, something will "click". My son-in-law, Dustin, became turned on to the Big Brother program and faithfully participates with his "little" brother. Maybe you are already "clicking" and now God calls you to greater spirituality. Again, that is between you and God.

By the way, if you are wondering what I ended up doing, you will be surprised. After much prayer, God revealed that the best thing I could do was to greet each person I meet at church and in other places with the warmth and love of Jesus. Many people who attend church and those out in the world are hurting, are lonely, ill, or the "prodigal son" returning. They need encouragement and I am someone to give it to them. We Christians tend to stake out our "territory" in church. If the service has already started, the pew seems full, and someone comes wanting to crowd into the pew, they get the "this is our spot and we're not moving" glare from fellow parishioners.

I imagine that the person coming in is my best friend and I want them to sit by me. I smile broadly and sometimes motion for them to come and sit by me and Lloyd. Brightens up their face and surprises them every time. I have met some wonderful people in this way. Your calling could be something as simple as that. It isn't always something world changing or grandiose, but something that changes one soul at a time. How very powerful you are—and God has chosen you. Thomas Merton also states that people have no idea what one saint can do and sanctity is stronger than all of hell. He further states that saints give themselves to the Lord, so that He may use His power through their smallest, and what seems to be insignificant ways, to save the world.[2] Say yes and watch it unfold.

August 28

Sometimes, I get weary following this holistic approach. There is so much to "do" to overcome illness and become in the pink of health. I watch people in a restaurant getting dishes dripping with cheese or eating fried chicken or chicken fried steak and it looks so tempting. Then, they order the gigantic piece of chocolate cake and my mouth really starts watering. Are they just a day away from some dreaded disease or a heart attack?

I'm glad we cook at home many nights so I don't see the temptation. I have switched to steel pots and pans since aluminum can leach into the foods, but food sometimes sticks in them. I miss my Teflon®! Ok, I can slap myself now and be thankful that I'm alive.

Help me, Lord, to crystallize, visualize, and materialize your plan for me to help others with this. **"It is I who will**

crystallize this for you. Continue on—everything you do is leading toward it. Be patient. Remember the unfolding of the flower. All my plans have their season and their time."

Getting Rid of Excess Metals

In every nutritional or healing book I have read, heavy metals prove to be a source of trouble. Mercury has been found in large quantities in people with symptoms of multiple sclerosis. Mercury is also the basis for many vaccines because it extends the shelf life. Controversy abounds about the relationship of mercury in vaccines to autism. I have begun to slowly get rid of my mercury fillings. My dentist is replacing them with porcelain and other non-metallic substances. According to Quillin in *BEATING CANCER WITH NUTRITION*, mercury poisoning causes a host of symptoms ranging from loss of memory to cancer. Mercury is used in coal-burning sites and used to coat seeds for planting! He stated that if one overlays a map of mercury pollution in the United Stated with locations of elevated incidents of cancer, they match.[3] Coincidence?

Copper has been in birth control pills, swimming pool chemicals used to kill algae that make the water turn green, and the most obvious, copper pipes carrying the water. Copper is needed by the body in small amounts. Lead is in pipes, water, old paint, gasoline fumes, and other sources. These metals were never meant to be taken into the body in the quantity in which they are currently ingested and they accumulate over time in the liver.

Aluminum has been associated with a host of diseased conditions, the most famous being Alzheimer's disease. I have disposed of all of my aluminum pans and any coated with a substance to make them "stick free". I purchased all stainless steel cookware. It is much more costly, but my return to health is worth it. Aluminum is in baking powder, so I have switched to alum-free baking powder and it works just as well. I don't even like to purchase drinks in aluminum cans. Aluminum is a major ingredient in deodorants. It is the ingredient that keeps underarms dry. I have changed deodorants to one that doesn't contain aluminum. It does have one disadvantage because the underarms don't remain dry. Exposure to one item containing aluminum may not cause immediate health problems but exposure to several of them or one used continuously could potentially be hazardous. The best advice is to limit the exposure to these items.

September 6

"You shall have all that you desire. It comes from me. Have faith. Continue to believe and all unfolds before you. It is like a royal carpet that slowly rolls open to reveal its beautiful colors. I am the carpet and I lay before you by the sacrifice I have made for you. And you have appreciated that sacrifice. Now, it is your turn to share in my glory. Hold on tight. We shall take a ride on the most beautiful carpet you have ever seen.

Love me unconditionally, for no conditions can be placed upon your Lord. I shower you with many gifts and blessings and I know you are grateful. I will show you how to use the gifts in ways that please me.

You will be ridiculed by some but I am teaching you how to overcome the ridicule just as I, the Christ, have overcome the world. Be patient. Look to me always. I am the supply. Amen" *I, the Lord, your God, teach you what is for your good, and lead you on the way you should go. (Isaiah 48:17)*

Giving and Receiving Unconditional Love

I have heard the term "unconditional love" but never pondered its meaning before now. God gives us unconditional love as evidenced by the crucifixion and death of Jesus. Jesus did not say, "I'll only go to the slaughter if people say they will appreciate it." Nor did God say, "I will only love you if you love me back." It is hard to grasp that He actually loves us no matter what we do or how we are. He always takes us back if we repent.

A difficult part of loving God or knowing him is to make that love free of "conditions". God has said that we are not allowed to say, "God, I'll only love you if you give me that brand new car I've been wanting," or "God, if you just let so-and-so love me, then I will worship and thank you." No conditions are to be placed on Him. He wants us to love Him as He loves us.

The first place to start practicing this is at home. For those of us with children, we love our children or our spouse unconditionally—or at least we should. We may not approve of what they do or how they act at all times, but we love them in spite of it all. The same thing applies with anyone you truly love. Lloyd may not always do things the way that I would, nor think like I do, but I love him anyway. And somehow, he loves me even though I rarely let him finish a sentence without interrupting. For many people, unconditional love is a foreign way of loving. Accept His unconditional love for you and tell Him so. Strive for an unconditional love of God and He will shower you with even more blessings because that pleases Him immensely. He created us to know and love Him.

September 13
Today was a HORRIBLE day. I heard dogs growling while upstairs. When I looked out the upstairs window into the back yard, I saw that the neighbor's two big dogs had dug a hole under the fence and come into our yard. They were shaking something back and forth and fighting over it when I realized to my absolute horror that it was a tiny gray and white kitten in their jaws! I screamed and ran breakneck speed down the stairs and out the back door. I made them drop it—its back was broken, one eye was bulging, and it had blood all over it. I gently knelt beside it as it turned its one good eye toward me, meowed weakly, and tried to move. It tried to clean itself as it lay dying. I knew there was no hope and I began to sob uncontrollably. I told it that I loved it as one of God's beautiful creatures and that it was not alone—that I was here. Five minutes later, it was dead. The horror of it all had been

unbelievable. That is why I don't watch those shows about wild kingdom on television.

Later, Lloyd and I buried the kitten and I prayed and cried. Then, we took the dogs back to their yard, and filled in and secured the hole in the fence. The neighbor wasn't home. Why, heavenly father? Why did I have to witness this? What was the purpose? Oh, my sorrow is great for all of your innocent creatures and children that die needlessly. They are so defenseless, just like that little kitten. The grief poured out of me like a river as I cried the rest of the day off and on. Oh, my Lord, help the innocents!

September 14

I've decided after yesterday that maybe I really don't like the number 13 after all. If I am the 13th disciple, then it's too tough of an assignment. Oh, Jesus, in reflecting, I realize that you, too, were an innocent who was crucified to achieve a greater good. Thank you for the unspeakable sufferings that you endured for our sake. **"There are people now experiencing unspeakable and unnecessary suffering all around the world. The ones of which I speak today are those that suffer at the hands of the medical profession. They are the innocents dying on the cross just as I did—crucified by their own people. Poisonous and barbaric treatments for any condition are not of me. Be the light."** Yes, Lord, I will gladly do as you ask but many people, especially the doctors and scientists, don't want to hear and refuse to listen or change their approach. **"Some seed WILL fall on fertile ground. Do not despair. Some of those who read this will awaken, rise up, and say, no more."** Praise and thanks to you, my one true God. *Blessed are your eyes because they see, and your ears because they hear. The seed sown on rich soil is the one who hears the word and understands it, who indeed bears fruit and yields a hundred or sixty or thirty fold. (Matthew 13:16,23)*

We Are All Innocents

I still do not understand why I have witnessed certain things and suffered other trials, but I do know that the Lord brings about a greater good. We do not "deserve" to suffer. It is not His will for us—ever. He only asked one to suffer and that was Jesus Christ. And a greater good came of it—victory over death, hope for mankind, and a new covenant, which brought about a new relationship with God. We are to focus on His mercy, forgiveness, goodness, and kindness. Does God know that we are going to suffer on this earth? Absolutely. Will we be able to see the greater good? Not always. Can we put an end to suffering? Most definitely. How will that occur? I can't answer that—we must leave the "how" to God and have trust in Him. We must pray to be awakened to all forms of truth that will work toward the elimination of the suffering of us all.

However, He has given me the task of awakening you and others to the horrors of treatments for disease. It is getting harder and harder for me to stand by while doctor after doctor recommends a treatment for a patient that he or she knows is absolutely going to hinder the patient and possibly kill him or her. Innocents like me and you who trust the medical profession are like lambs being led to the slaughter. Whenever I hear the term "radical treatment" or "aggressive treatment," I cringe at the hidden underlying meaning. The hidden meaning is "This is probably going to kill you, but we are going to try it anyway for the sake of science."

I came across two interesting interviews of Dr. Nicholas Gonzalez, a physician in New York, who treats patients with serious diagnoses using alternative methods. The interview was posted at *www.the-moneychanger.com.*[4] (See bibliography for specific article addresses.) and leads one to deduce why chemotherapy and radiation often lead to more tumors later on instead of curing cancer. He cited a long lost book by Casper Blond, an English surgeon, entitled *THE LIVER AND CANCER*. The most fascinating information in the article, to me, is that one of the primary functions of the liver is to remove toxins. When the liver becomes "full" of toxins, or damaged, it can no longer function optimally. What does the body do? It forms a tumor. The purpose of the tumor is to absorb more toxins and act as a second or third or fourth liver. When Dr. Johanna Budwig, of Germany, performed research and analyzed soft tumors, she found that they often contained hydrogenated oils. The tumor is trying to protect the body from these foreign substances that can't be used by the body. The body actually forms a protective layer around the substance to try and seal it off. This explained the process and helped me tremendously.[5]

Herein lies the problem with chemotherapy. We have a trusting "innocent" who comes to the doctor with an already overloaded liver and then the doctor, either because he or she believes in the traditional treatment or in order to protect him or herself from getting accused of not providing "Standard of Care," orders chemotherapy or radiation, or both. Chemotherapy drugs are highly toxic chemicals. Upon administration of the drugs, an overloaded liver becomes super overloaded, the toxins possibly kill the growing tumors (many times they don't), and definitely kill the growing red and white cells along with many other growing and regenerating cells that the body needs.

For a short while, the person might be pronounced free and clear and told they are in "remission", but the new tumors are already forming to handle the megatoxic overload of chemicals now circulating in the body. The liver's immune ability is destroyed. The person gets sicker and sicker instead of better. What is wrong with this picture? We must wake up and realize what is happening to the innocents! Why does the medical profession allow this to go on? Why do insurance companies go along with this expensive treatment? It costs them tons of money each year and with more and more people getting diagnosed with cancer, the expenses will exponentially continue to grow.....like an unchecked tumor....a definite pun intended here.

According to Dr. Gonzalez, a friend of his stated that the National Institutes of Health, which oversees cancer research, is full of highly intelligent scientists who are constantly competing with each other. Egos are at stake, as well as government job security. Mediocrity has taken over. They will call the media to report a new cancer drug even if it is not effective or only minimally effective in order to secure more government funding. For example, a chemotherapy drug, Gemzar® (which is the one they gave me), was approved by the FDA for pancreatic cancer.

If the patient did not take Gemzar®, he or she lived four and a half months. If they took Gemzar®, they lived five and a half months. It helped with pain, but only temporarily—all of that money and misery for a one month extension of life. Another case was the approval of Interleukin-2. It was just as successful as a 'placebo' (an inactive substance given to part of the patients as a control) in treating kidney cancer, which was only 6 percent of the time. It costs around $200,000 for a complete round and yet, the FDA approved it.[6] If presented with ideas that work, scientists and doctors stifle those ideas or ridicule them, even if the alternative treatments could save lives. Unfortunately the scientists do not always have the interests of the 'innocents' in mind. *They sacrificed their sons and their daughters to the demons. They shed innocent blood, the blood of their sons and daughters, whom they sacrificed to the idols of Canaan, and the land was desecrated by their blood. They defiled themselves by what they did; by their deeds they prostituted themselves. (Psalm 106:37-39)*

I read a very disconcerting article in *Life Extension Magazine*, by the founder, William Faloon[7]. He pointed out several problems with the FDA. The current practices of the FDA have allowed dangerous drugs to be put on the market, two examples being Ketek® and Paxil®. Ketek®, given to infants, causes toxicities to the heart, eyes, and liver, while Paxil® has caused a 6.7 times increase in suicidal behavior. The FDA allows drugs like these and then denounces holistic items with no known toxicity. Dr. Gonzalez also has a website, *www.dr-gonzalez.com* for you to view.

The medical profession has adopted these substandard treatments which violate the Hippocratic Oath; "To please no one will I prescribe a deadly drug..." Antibiotics are prescribed that damage the liver and do not always work effectively. Doctors get caught up in the same type of rivalry and fear of losing patients and the innocents suffer. I listened to a cassette tape made by a doctor who stated that a woman came to him with a sick baby. He told her to feed the baby diluted unpasteurized goat's milk. The woman eventually did as he requested and the baby became healthy and vibrant. The following week, he received a call from the child's angry doctor accusing Dr. Robbins of trying to steal his patient, even though he'd been unable to help the child after many visits. What about what is best for the patient?

In her book, *Outsmart Your Cancer: Alternative Non-Toxic Treatments That Work*, by Tanya Pierce, the lives and work of several people, including medical doctors, were discussed. Besides Rene Caisse with her Essiac tea formula, several others stood out. One was Dr. Max Gerson, a renowned doctor from Germany who had tremendous success with diet and detoxification for a number of illnesses, including cancer. Without going into great detail, he was literally kicked out of the medical society and his methods were labeled by the AMA (American Medical Association) as a "false notion." The information he presented in medical papers was not accepted by the JAMA (Journal of the AMA) and the information was, in effect, kept from the public. He tried the National Cancer Institute and offered them five success cases. They wanted 25. He provided them with the 25 and then they wanted 125. The NCI never evaluated them.[8] *Hail shall sweep away the refuge of lies, and waters shall flood the hiding place. Your covenant with death shall be canceled and your pact with the nether world shall not stand. (Isaiah 28:17-18)*

God does not want this. It is not natural. God does not want us to suffer. We should not have to suffer violently to heal. Healing should be a natural, gently unfolding process. Keep this thought uppermost in your mind. Neither you, nor anyone you love, deserves or needs to suffer. God help us innocents. I cry out to you. Hear the voice of your people. *While from behind, a voice shall sound in your ears: This is the way: walk in it. (Isaiah 30: 21)*

Heavenly Pearls of Wisdom

Walk the path for God. Your story is unique just like you are and it is important to God's mission.

God chose you. He didn't make a mistake or get mixed up. YOU are the one.

Strive for perfect love. God will help you love him unconditionally.

Replace heavy metals. For every metal in your life, there is a healthier substitute. Start with your cooking utensils.

God does not want you to suffer. Put those old beliefs behind you. God wants you in the condition of perfection to do his will.

10
Mercy of the Lord

September 26
Today is my 59th birthday. Hallelujah! I am very blessed to be here and in what I consider good health! We had the resources and time to take a short trip to Freeport, Grand Bahamas with Andraya and Derek and I enjoyed it all with renewed appreciation for the beautiful water, the wonderful people, and feeling free. We signed up to go snorkeling on a 54-foot Catamaran, and as it turned out, we were the only 4 on the entire boat plus the crew of 2! It was fun to pretend that it was a private charter with our own captain! Thank you, thank you, thank you, Lord! I love your beautiful Caribbean. Only you could have created something so magnificent and full of beautiful fish and living sea plants and animals. I wish many blessings upon the people there. Amen.

October 1
Another month is gone. It is hard to imagine that they go so fast and I thank the Lord for each and every day. I heard the Lord say these words to me at least 3 times, **"Receive ye the Holy Spirit."** I felt such joy and peace in my heart and soul. I don't yet know what the ramifications of that are, but for now I am going to enjoy the peace and joy that it brought.

October 2

Another day! Praise be to God! I read today, in a book called *THE MASTER SPEAKS*, by Joel Goldsmith, that when you make contact with the Lord and really believe in Him and feel His presence that all you need unfolds before you. Problems are solved without much trouble, success follows, the Spirit goes before you and attracts to you all that is necessary for your unfolding.[1] Oh, Lord, I thank you for all of this. YOU are all that I need. But for whatever else you provide that I need, I thank you. I know that you are unlimited. I love watching the beautiful carpet unroll before me. How great is your name. Amen.

October 4

I picked up a highlighter to highlight some passages in my Bible and I noticed that the marker said "refillable." This one word actually caused me to pause and reflect. This word describes our life. When we feel "spent," it is the grace of God that "refills" us. We probably don't see it or feel it, but it surely happens. It occurs even faster if we call upon Him. Then He said, **"Call upon me and I will refresh you. I will fill you with healing waters of grace like a health spa for the soul. My spirit fills you to overflowing so that grace can be shared with others. Let it flow. Give it away and I refill you. I am the infinite supply."** Lord, thank you for refilling me and for your insights. They are always so profound and way beyond my thinking or intellectualizing. Fill me with your loving grace this day that I might share you with souls longing to reconnect with you. Thank you for your abundance in all areas. Amen.

October 8

I still get a headache the next day after I go to the clinic for a treatment. I will be so happy when my body becomes detoxified enough that this no longer happens. And I know it will.

> I am regenerating from the inside out. My liver is getting rid of 59 years' worth of toxins of various types. It's too bad we can't really see our liver filling up with these or we would not wait to detoxify until it gets overwhelmed and we get diseases. I'd heard about detoxification but just didn't think it would ever apply to me. Now I realize that it applies to everybody.

Detoxification is Crucial

I saved the discussion of this part of my treatment for later because it usually either turns people off or scares them off if they don't fully comprehend its importance. But it is one of the three most crucial elements to physical healing. The first is to change the diet and nutrition, the second is to add supplements, and the third is detoxification. First of all, there are certainly many ways of detoxifying the body. I received colonic hydrotherapy treatments at the clinic which are very effective. However, one of the most effective at-home ways of detoxifying the liver is touted by the alternative and natural healing practitioners and sometimes condemned by the medical community or others who do not understand it fully. I am talking about coffee enemas. Yes, coffee and enema in the same sentence and they are actually called "high enemas."

What is a coffee enema? One brews up a pot of regular caffeinated coffee (organic is best) and dilutes it to 2 quarts. This is placed in an enema bag. The person lies down with the bag hanging higher than the body to allow the liquid to flow by gravity into the entire large intestine. The coffee is held for 5-8 minutes, and then expelled. When the colon is entirely filled, it actually triggers the smooth muscles of the intestines to contract very strongly as if a person is having a bowel movement. Therefore, do not fall for the false claim that a person gets dependent upon the enema. If one stops the enemas, normal movements will resume in about 2-3 days, assuming a normal diet is eaten.

High enemas are not to be confused with "low" enemas, which are used to relieve constipation. Low enemas can cause dependency because only a small amount of liquid is used and only to fill the rectum. Low enemas should only be used sparingly.

Coffee contains compounds, one of them being caffeine, that actually stimulate the liver to release many of its long-held toxins. According to the book, *Prescription for Nutritional Healing*, by Dr. James Balch and Phyllis Balch, C.N.C., high coffee enemas additionally stimulate the gall bladder to release toxins and they recommend a coffee temperature of around 99°F. The high coffee enema is also used for the relief of pain.[2] Dr. Nicholas Gonzalez, the physician of whom I spoke earlier, uses them extensively in his practice and he and his staff routinely partake.[3] Yes, it sounds awful. People will try to say it is dangerous. However, they have been done since the days of the Pharaohs in Egypt. Until the 1970's, when it was supposedly removed for space reasons, one could find it in the Merck Manual for medicine.

They were used extensively by Jethro Kloss, a famed healer in the 1930's. His book, *Back to Eden*, talks of all sorts of high and low enemas used for healing.[4] I personally know people who work at the Holistic Health Care Center in Boerne, Texas, that have been doing them faithfully every day for anywhere from 8-20 years and are in excellent health. Many people are able to get off of medications they have been on for years. It is worth the effort.

Why can't we just drink more coffee? Alas! If only that were the answer. The first reason is that coffee in the stomach mixes with stomach acid which changes its composition. Secondly, drinking coffee by mouth actually causes the liver duct to close up and not release toxins. Drinking coffee in excess also makes the body too acidic, setting it up for diseased conditions.

As we recall, when the liver is overloaded, the body tries to rid the blood of waste through the skin, kidneys, lungs, and any other portal it can. If those systems also become overwhelmed, the body then creates a second liver, a tumor, to absorb the toxins. When that tumor becomes overburdened, the body creates more tumors. And we know the rest of the story. Therefore, the key to recovery is to detoxify the liver. I use 6 tablespoons of regular coffee to 6 cups of water and dilute it, after brewing, to 2 quarts. Additionally, everything in contact with the body must be thoroughly cleaned afterward with a good antibacterial soap. At first, it may be difficult to retain the full two quarts because the colon is full of waste material. (Those experiencing any colon or rectal bleeding or ulcers should not use this method.) In the beginning, I did them two times a day to get rid of all chemotherapy residue and past exposure to toxins that extremely overwhelmed my liver. I can tell you that within one to two weeks of starting the detoxification process, I felt infinitely better in terms of energy, pain relief, and over all well-being.

I talked with a registered dietician and told her of the benefits of the coffee enemas. She immediately said in reply, "Our bodies have natural methods of eliminating toxins and waste so we don't need to resort to extraordinary measures." And my response was, "In a former life that was true, but we have an extraordinary amount of pesticides and herbicides in our soil, food, and water. More people are getting sicker every day. Combine that with the amount of chemicals we absorb into our bodies and you can see why the liver was never designed to handle that much toxicity."

I could tell that she did not accept my words, but I have to face reality. It is time for the lies and burying the head in the sand to stop. My hope is that people wake up to this.

The pesticide and herbicide industry, along with the drug industry, try their darnedest to keep the truth from the masses. Look at the Erin Brockovich story. The whole town was being poisoned by a chemical called Hexavalent Chromium leaching into the soil. The gas and electric company responsible not only denied it but tried to prevent the truth from being exposed by ordering an employee to shred documents that spoke of high levels of the carcinogenic chemical in their holding ponds.[6] *For we have made lies our refuge, and in falsehood we have found a hiding place. (Isaiah 28:15)*

The wonderful other benefit is that I no longer have headaches like I had before. I dreamed of the day when I would be free of migraine headaches. During my last year of working full time as an educational administrator, I woke up with a headache almost every day. I spent many days pretending that I was feeling well. Little did I know that the headaches were a sign of toxic overload. Headaches mean that the blood is full of toxins and the liver is unable to remove them in a timely manner. The headaches are gone. Thanks be to God.

You will want to do your own research. There are herbs that will do the same thing, although more slowly. An excellent, easy to take herb for the liver is Silymarin (commonly called Milk Thistle). I take 40 drops per day of a low-alcohol tincture. I put it in a hot liquid every morning and drink it up. Even if one were just to do this, it would be extremely beneficial and the liver would thank the person. There are detoxification "kits" that one can purchase. Buyer beware. Some of these products do absolutely nothing and how would one know unless one felt better immediately as a result? Check every product out as thoroughly as possible.

Juicing fresh vegetables, as mentioned earlier, is another way to help the detoxification process. My herbalist also recommends squeezing the juice of one lemon in distilled water, adding a pinch of red pepper flakes and drinking the mixture right down. The question is whether or not some of these other methods can detoxify a "diseased" body fast enough to overcome the illness. This is something you must read and pray about to choose what is best for your body or that of a loved one.

October 21

I went out to feed the birds and discovered a beautiful male cardinal who could not fly for some reason and was quite flustered and scared. Oh, my heart became so troubled to see one of God's marvelous creatures incapacitated and vulnerable to predators. Also, the hawks have been using our yard as a hunting ground lately. What could I do? Who could I call? My mind became frantic. He hid himself as best he could under my lantana plant but with that bright red color, he was definitely not camouflaged.

I went in the house and prayed fervently. "Oh, Lord, if we are a part of you and you are a part of us, then, as your disciples, we have the power to heal. Let your glory shine forth and allow me to heal this little bird. I need this because my faith is small. Heal the little bird. Help me believe." I returned out to the yard and the bird was gone. I checked everywhere and checked for a bunch of feathers to indicate that something had "gotten" him but there were none. I checked the neighbor's yards on either side of me and behind. I believe he actually flew off! O, sigh of sighs. Thank you, Lord. You are so merciful. Amen.

November 18

"Focus on my mercy. Focus on my goodness. Man would have you focus on all that is evil. You are surrounded by those thoughts. You hear it everyday. Release those thoughts. They are harmful to the spirit. Embrace the light. My light shines forth always, but men put a cloak over their faces. That is the veil of which the Bible speaks. I have not placed the veil over man's eyes. He has done so himself."

But, Lord, what about those who are unrepentant? Do you have mercy on them also? **"I deal with those in due season. I give each person many times and circumstances to repent. I alone determine when the time is up. It is mercy that prevails always."** Oh, my Lord, thank you for the mercy you have shown me. I ask for continued mercy on me and all of us. **"It is granted."**

November 23

Today, while I was in church I clearly heard words from the Lord. Sometimes I marvel at how all of this came about. But I love the Lord taking over my thoughts. Lord, you can have all of me—my thoughts, my body, my soul, my strength, my days, my minutes, my seconds, my spirit—you can have them all to serve your higher purpose. **"My mercy surrounds you like a cloak, my love penetrates you like a sword, and my grace flows through you like a channel from the ocean. This manifests as goodness. And so it is with all people. Impart this message. Tell them to offer it as a simple prayer to me, their Lord.**

"Lord, cloak me in your mercy.
Pierce me with your love.
Pour your grace through me. Amen."

It is so simple, yet so powerful and inclusive. Say it often in every situation." Yes, Lord, I hear and obey. As our thanksgiving holiday approaches, I remain thankful to you for everything.

God's Mercy Freely Given

During church services I hear the word "mercy" used all of the time. In fact, I think many of us have gotten so used to hearing the word that it really has no real depth of meaning for us any more. God's mercy is IMPORTANT! He wants to cover us in it. Having mercy means that whatever the judgment could be in terms of our actions, thoughts, or attitudes, God overlooks quite a bit and keeps working with us. *But God, being rich in mercy, because of his great love with which He loved us, even when we were dead in our transgressions, made us alive together with Christ. (Ephesians 2:4-5)*

Even on the cross, when the sinner next to him repented, Jesus had immense mercy on him and that guy had been a criminal most of his life! He'd been a "career criminal" who said he deserved his punishment from the Romans. *And He (Jesus) said to him, 'Truly I say to you, today you shall be with me in paradise. (Luke 23:43)*

We must repent of anything that offends the Divine Being. Most of the things we do, we are well aware of. If you steal something from someone, you know you have done wrong. But, we all do things that hurt ourselves or others unintentionally. Repent of those things too. Repent of wrong thoughts, wrong attitudes, wrong actions, wrong inactions and mercy will flow like Niagara Falls. Mercy also comes from God to us who aren't repentant, but our hearts are hardened at that point and not willing to receive it when offered. *Then he (Jesus) began to denounce the cities in which most of his miracles were done, because they did not repent. (Matthew 11:20)*

Feeling worthy to accept mercy is another stumbling block for us. None of us are worthy of anything. We are only worthy because we have part of the Divine in us. That, along with a contrite heart, makes us worthy of the mercy of the Lord. Therefore, in order for God's mercy to be effective in achieving growth in our spirit, we pray for mercy, accept that mercy, and be thankful for it. When we accept mercy with a thankful heart, we behold a great healing process in our body. Once our spirit stands erect again, so does our body. *For indeed he was sick to the point of death, but God had mercy on him, and not on him only, but also on me, so that I would not have sorrow upon sorrow. (Philippians 2:27)*

Thomas Merton, in *The Seven Storey Mountain*, states that when holy people (saints) remember their sins, they do not concentrate on the sins, but remember the mercy of God. This turns their past misdeeds into a present cause for joy and glorifies God.[6]

November 25

I prayed, "Lord, thank you for your words to me and your words in the Bible for all people." His reply was, **"My words in the Book have meaning for you and the words I give to you are also for all. All people need to believe in my love. All need to believe in my mercy. Those terms have been tossed about as though casually tossing a ball to and fro**

without any cares or contemplation. Love and mercy have meaning in every life. My love and mercy are shown to people in ways of which they are not aware. They are asleep to the world of the spirit.

Awakening occurs for each, in time. Unfortunately, for some, it happens with an event that saddens. I do not 'send' these events. They, too, unfold as part of the earthly existence. Then, people cry out to me and when my answer comes, they actually feel my love and mercy in their very soul, as you have done. Do not take my love and mercy lightly. Feel them and impart them to others. That is my commandment. Those who do this experience great peace and healing in their own souls. Amen"

November 26

Mary, my cousin's wife, called from California. My cousin John went into surgery to unclog his carotid artery and right after surgery, suffered a stroke. They would not normally have known this but his doctor insisted that he be somewhat conscious throughout the procedure. They kept having him squeeze a ball with each hand. All of a sudden, he could not feel his hand on the left side and could not squeeze the ball. Immediately, they took him back to surgery, discovered a clot right above his ear, reopened the incision, and went in and took out the clot. At this point he is unable to move his left side after coming out of the surgery.

Mary asked me to pray for him and of course, I said that I would. However, I told her, "Mary, we must picture him as whole, perfect, and complete. He is made in the image of God." Later that evening I prayed earnestly to the Lord and I prayed the simple prayer he had just taught me. "Lord, cloak John in your mercy, pierce him with your love, and pour your grace through him." I sent grace and healing to him and to her. And I prayed for myself. "Lord, if you really wish for me to heal others, show me, by his healing, that this IS possible. Help me—not I, but by Christ that is within me."

The next day, Mary e-mailed that John could now move his arms, legs, and all other parts and was bugging the doctor to go home! There will be some physical therapy involved, but it sure beats being paralyzed on one side for the remainder of his days. Thanks be to God—the Lord is kind and merciful! He can return to his normal life and play more golf, too!

How much more proof do I need of God's mercy? No more proof. I know that His mercy surrounds us if we just claim it and look for it. I hear more stories like this the more aware that I become. May he open all of our eyes to His mercy and lift the veil. Pray for God's mercy, repent, believe that you are worthy of it, receive the mercy of the Lord, and wait for continued healing of anything mental, spiritual, and physical.

December 12

I went to the doctor today for a bladder infection. I will take an antibiotic, even though I don't want to. I have been unable to beat it with natural methods.

He is the same doctor who gave me the bad news of cancer two years ago. He asked how I was doing and I told him that, except for the bladder infection, I was doing absolutely fantastic—that every ailment I'd ever come to him with was gone. He asked how I'd done it. So, I explained the entire holistic program. I also told him that I had visited another doctor who had explained to me why no doctor can embrace this approach.

Immediately, he said, "We physicians are bound by a STANDARD of CARE that absolutely must be based on scientific, proven research. Has your clinic done scientific research to know and prove that these methods really work?" I told him no, they had not, because they are too busy taking care of patients! He then said that research is very expensive and that drug companies are pretty much the only ones who have the money to do it. The asparagus industry is not going to fund a study on its role in helping with cancer. He stressed that what I was doing was not proven and had no research behind it. He didn't even feel comfortable making dietary recommendations to his patients without research.

I was so disheartened. What, O Lord, has happened to us as a society? The doctor said that if he made 'unproven' recommendations and then they didn't work, that he could get sued for not providing the STANDARD of CARE, and could lose his license. Say what? The medical profession has itself frightened to do anything! He is a victim of his own colleagues!

As a nation, we are getting sicker and sicker. I cry out to you, God. Save us! Save us from ourselves! We have come no further in cancer treatment than we were 30 years ago. The more this nation focuses on "cancer" instead of prevention and change, the more we will see. When we focus on something, we bring more of it to ourselves. We need to focus on wellness, well being, and wholeness. It's not just for the "health nuts." It's a matter of life or early death.

Help reveal the TRUTH! Father, let your power be seen. And remove the fear in me that the doctor unknowingly tried to instill by telling me that I don't know how many people have died at the clinic or how many times they are unsuccessful.

We patients, as well as others, meet with the director once a week. I've been there. I've gotten to know many of the patients. I DO have an idea of how many they have lost and why. Most are brought to them way too late, after chemotherapy and radiation or other treatments have destroyed them and they are given up for dead. Others have no support from family members and end up leaving too soon after treatment begins. I have seen many healings and my friend Grace is one of them. Others are "still in progress". Renew my faith, Lord. Help me and others stand against Goliath. I desperately need you now. Hear me again—answer me again. Amen.

December 15
Lloyd took me to the emergency room with a rapid heart beat of 160 beats per minute and a blood pressure of 212/100! It came on suddenly and lasted for several hours. Oh, it felt like I was dying and I prayed a lot. It was absolutely a horrible feeling. I cannot describe it adequately here.

The interviewing doctor, upon learning that I had been diagnosed with ovarian cancer, stated that after chemotherapy, they often see women in there with blood clots in the lungs! Isn't that just great! He also said that chemotherapy may damage heart tissue and produce Paroxysmal Atrial Tachycardia (cells that cause the heart to beat too fast). So, they were going to run a bunch of tests.

I am appalled that when I go to the pharmacist to pick up any prescription, the pharmacist advises me or gives me a paper with the information of side effects and so on. BUT, when they gave me chemotherapy, there was no information AT ALL provided about side effects, nor any other information. I don't even know what kind of dosage I was given, even though the doctor decided to reduce it after the first treatment. Why do they keep us in the dark? None of my friends received any information either. What is up with that? How is that possible? Where is the STANDARD of CARE there? So many of the chemotherapy drugs produce serious kidney, heart, liver, nerve damage or a different type of cancer or leukemia which often lead to life threatening situations in themselves! Why aren't people complaining about this? How do the drug companies get away with that?

The emergency room doctor also said that the antibiotic I was on could cause anxiety. I had taken this antibiotic many times in the past. What next?

After lots of tests and many hours later, the hospital said that the only thing they could find was a low blood potassium level, to get with my primary doctor about it, and sent me home. That was it! They didn't even give me any potassium!

It makes no sense to me. My pulse had dropped some and my blood pressure was not as high when I walked out of the ER.

The next day, I called Melissa at the clinic and she said that if I had called her, she could have helped me. She said that many times antibiotics deplete the body of potassium and other minerals. This causes the rapid heart beat and can cause the blood pressure to go haywire. So, she increased my potassium supplements, adjusted some other supplements and soon all was back to normal! What a scare! Now, I will be very hesitant to take an antibiotic.

Lord, I pray that I be strengthened and do not give in to fear with every incident. I love you, Lord. Be here with me. Help me through the "gray days". Amen.

December 21

Today, the Lord spoke. **"Listen with your heart, Diana. Many people think that my message comes in ways they expect. Look for the unexpected. I do not speak to the head as the rest of the world does, but to the heart. I gave man a heart that pumps the lifeblood as a symbol of my spiritual 'lifeblood' that should flow in all of your spiritual veins and arteries. And, just as blood recirculates—leaves the heart and returns to the heart full of oxygen—so it is with grace.**

The grace and love that you send out returns to you even more. All things on earth are symbols of my 'spiritual laws'. I will continue to reveal them to you as you have sought wisdom. Therefore, let all grace flow through your heart and let your heart have 'ears', just as the body hears its own heartbeat.

I speak to the heart in many circumstances of ordinary days. Be alert for all that occurs, the people you encounter. Show them the love of my sacred heart. Every chance encounter is not by chance. Each one is an opportunity for you to speak my love with your heart. Listen with your

heart and speak with your heart. Amen." *For this people's heart has become calloused; they hardly hear with their ears, and they have closed their eyes. Otherwise they might see with their eyes, hear with their ears, understand with their hearts and turn, and I would heal them. (Matthew 13:15)*

In *The Seven Storey Mountain*, one sentence by Merton particularly struck me. I read it shortly after this message. He said, "They (the Trappist Monks) had been transformed into Him by the pure and absolute humility of their hearts."[7] In every circumstance, if we have a humble heart, and are receptive to grace, we are being slowly transformed. Transformed into what? Transformed into Him. What a revelation. *...what we shall be has not yet been revealed. We do know that when it is revealed we shall be like him, for we shall see him as he is. (1 John 3:2)*

December 23
It is almost Christmas.

Dear Jesus, I ask that you continue to reveal your truths of the kingdom to me. As I become aware of each truth, help me to believe it and to internalize it. Then, help me to live it. May I manifest it to others and share it with those who are ready for it. For your glory. Amen.

I received my blood work from the hospital. It's been one and a half years since chemotherapy and my white cell count is STILL working its way back up to normal. It is now at 3.3 (normal is 4-10). Almost there! My platelets are also STILL working their way up. They are at 126 and normal is at least 150. Chemotherapy is so devastating. If only people knew the truth. Oh, help us all, my Lord. Reveal the truth and do not let it fall on deaf ears. Amen. *In your majesty ride forth victoriously in behalf of truth, humility, and righteousness; let your right hand display awesome deeds. (Psalm 45:4)*

December 27
I had a wonderful, fantastic Christmas. Both daughters were here, along with Dustin and Derek. We went to my ex-husband's house (Bob) for Christmas day (which is amazing considering that most people don't even talk to an ex-spouse) and did our own gift exchange on the 26th. I talked with my mom and dad also. All is well. Thank you, Lord, for so much. Compared to where we were a year ago with my mom having a stroke on Christmas Eve, this is an especially beautiful Christmas. You are so gracious and merciful, God. Amen…Amen.

January 1
Happy another year!

"All that I have is yours. I keep nothing from you. Only you keep it from yourself. My kingdom is here for all to partake of. They must pray and wait patiently—then act when it is time to act—at my direction. Many people worry that they will not know what to do. If they have asked me for help and guidance, I will send them the Holy Spirit to put the 'knowing' within their very being.

It is often so subtle that they do not recognize it as my gentle touch. They wait for a big revelation. I feed them in small nourishing ways because the total revelation of all they cannot handle. If one eats a meal too quickly, one becomes too full and gets ill. But, if one eats slowly, chewing, digesting, and appreciating each morsel, they become pleasantly full and can now go about My work. I feed you and others all that is needed as it is needed. Accept it graciously and thankfully. Amen"

Lord, I ask that you continue to feed me with your nourishing grace as I am able to handle it. Sometimes I think that I don't do enough, or that I'm developing too slowly spiritually, but your words encourage me. I must take each new (or not so new, but maybe forgotten) lesson and recognize it (awaken to it), meditate on it (chew it), internalize it (digest it), and make it part of me (accept it graciously).

At other times, I heed all that your word says while I am in communion with you and then five minutes after I return to the real world, I instantly forget it. **"Ask for my grace to not only fill you but to sustain you—remember, it IS possible with me. Go about your day with my sustaining grace. Amen"**

Truths to Be Learned

In all that happens to us, both joyful and sorrowful, there is a truth of the heavenly kingdom that is to be learned. That truth is different for each one of us. I am sharing with you the truths that were revealed to me. They are good for all to know but there are some others that you are learning as you live your story or someone you know lives theirs. It's kind of like a fable, in which there is a moral to be learned. That's what life is like—a series of fables, each with a moral. *Guide me in your truth, and teach me, for you are God my savior, and my hope is in you all day long. (Psalm 25:5)*

Truths are given to us as we can truly internalize them. We can repeat truths all day such as God is good, God is merciful, I am loved, and so forth, but until they are written on our humble hearts, they remain external to us and just words. Remember, we are becoming Him through this internalization process. *Surely you desire truth in your inner parts; you teach me wisdom in the inmost place. (Psalm 51:6)*

Think about the twelve apostles. They did not get it right away. They were slow to understand. They didn't get it after hearing Jesus preach and seeing his miracles. They still didn't totally get it when he was crucified, nor when he rose from the dead. When did they get it? They finally got it when the Holy Spirit descended upon them in the upper room. They then internalized and lived it. Once they lived it, they preached it to others. *I tell you the truth, whoever accepts anyone I send accepts me; and whoever accepts me accepts the one who sent me. (John 13:20)*

Jesus spoke much about the truth. In fact, he said, "I tell you the truth" quite often as he spoke. He had many truths to teach and not much earthly time in which to do it. One of the apostles, Thomas, bemoaned to Jesus that they didn't know where he was going so how would they know the way? *And Jesus answered, 'I am the way and the truth and the life. No one comes to the father except through me.' (John 14:6)*

Once you learn the truth, internalize it, and try to teach it, others may not be so receptive. As Joel Goldsmith states in *The Master Speaks*, "The men and women of the world are afraid to learn about spiritual truth, because they know that once they have been touched by the Spirit, never again could they do the same things in business, or their home life, never again could they be the same to their families."[8] The truth will do its own work. I am waiting for the truth to work in the medical community and insurance companies. When it does, it will save the insurance companies lots of money and lessen human suffering. They need to pay for alternative treatments rather than only traditional ones. I have faith. *I tell you the truth, we speak of what we know, and we testify to what we have seen, but still you people do not accept our testimony. (John 3:11)*

We must pray with a humble heart to be taught the truths. When you become humble and receptive, you will be granted the truths of God and *...you will know the truth and the truth will make you free. (John 8:32)* What will you be free of? You will be free of disease, free of fear, free of your old ways, free of your old self. You will not be the same person and you will be changing. And change is not a bad thing if it is for your greater good and the glory of God. You are becoming Him.

Heavenly Pearls of Wisdom

You must detoxify your body. Your future freedom from disease depends on it. Find a way, embrace it, and be faithful to it.

God's mercy abounds. You are surrounded by it, cloaked in it. Claim it and be healed.

Listen with your heart. Sometimes our head doesn't always "get it", but our heart will. We often hear that we will know in our heart. It is true.

You are learning truths. God is teaching them to you one by one with every circumstance. Internalize them and teach them to others.

11
Beyond the Earthly Senses

January 4
I caught some sort of cold or flu. I had a fever and felt miserable. Then, the cedar pollen from the north hit and my body reacted to that also. My nose was non-stop running and now I have a sinus infection. What is going on with me? Last year at this time, I was perfectly fine and my allergies, I thought, were gone forever. Now, they have returned again.

Does this mean my immune system isn't working like it should? Am I regressing? Is this the evil one trying to come against me as a fake power? I haven't been able to listen to the Lord. My receivers have been out of tune or something. My body is definitely out of balance.

Lord, I know you are there even though I can't hear you. You are part of me. Otherwise, I would be mere dust and have no being. Help me in my distress of body, soul, and spirit. Only you can put things back in balance.

"I am indeed here. Believe in me. Do not fret. I have not abandoned you. Be patient. Love others. Even a loving thought directed to them helps each one turn to my love. Peace be with you."

January 5
We went to a Christmas concert even though it is after Christmas. The orchestra had a delayed tour. That was really neat, but I was so congested that no one wanted to be near me. I called Melissa at the clinic and she has me doing sinus washes with a product called NeilMed™. I am also taking oregano and Echinacea. I am getting better but why not faster?

"Diana, you must not react according to how you feel. The use of the five senses will deceive you. The senses are NOT your reality. For those that are ill, no matter what they see or feel, they must not give in to that. My kingdom is beyond feeling or seeing. Focus on only me—my attributes of harmony, balance, mercy, and love. Know beyond a shadow of a doubt that they exist above the plane of the 5 senses. If those who are ill focus on how they feel and what they see, they deny me and my power.

This allows them to give in to the earthly senses and can come to no good—only more of the same. The 5 senses are merely signals of what goes on. They are not what you should live by nor what you should give in to."

Then, what are we to do, Lord? What do we do when we feel pain or see disease?

"Give thanks that you know me, your Lord, and that I know you. Be thankful that I am part of you. *Beloved, let us love one another, because love is of God; everyone who loves is begotten by God and knows God. (I John 4:7)* **Ask to let me shine through all feeling and seeing. Ask me to let you spiritually feel me in every cell of your body. Breathe deeply and ask to feel the Holy Spirit in your breath. See, in your mind, my light, heaven, piercing each cell in your body to drive out the darkness.** *Therefore, let us cast off the works of darkness and let us put on the armor of light. (Romans 13:12)* **Do this much each day. Give in to me. Give in to my light—my power—not to your earthly senses. They were given to you to use but not to live by."**

January 8
O Lord, I don't seem to be getting any better. Is my problem physical? Is it mental? Is it spiritual? Something is eating at me on the inside. I feel impatient. Where am I on the continuum Lord?

"How peaceful are you? If you are at great peace in all circumstances, then my kingdom is yours. What is impatience? It is the opposite of peace. What is peace? It is a gift of the Holy Spirit.

Ask for this gift. Ask. I wait patiently for you to ask. Ask and it shall be done to you. Emotionalism connected with earthly things works against peace. Pray for yourself and others. Peace be with you. My peace I give to you. But, you must accept it. Accept it and it is yours. If you lose it, pray to regain it. Pray. I am always here. Even a single prayer—Lord, grant me peace—is heard. You must remember who you are in all matters. You are of me. No one can take that from you. Cherish me. Amen"

January 11
Today is the exact day two years ago that I was diagnosed with life threatening cancer. I am so happy to be here, alive and doing well. I will be grateful even more when I can write that it has been 10 or 20 years so that it will no longer be even a faint memory. This has been the most difficult journey of my life, but in it, I have found joy for I have begun to know the Lord more fully. All glory to you, my Lord and savior.

January 14
Now, I have a cough and am losing my voice. What is going on? Why am I not healing? I am still sneezing up a storm with the cedar pollen. I am trying not to get frightened. This is discouraging. I am taking Vitamin C, herbs, and doing nasal washes. I am trying to ignore the 5 senses, but they are pretty insistent. Lord, help me to overcome this adversity. What a way to start a new year.

January 23
I almost got rid of the sinus infection and now it has come back with a renewed vengeance. My voice is worse now and the cedar pollen is still trying to get me. This is getting ridiculous. Lord, it is so difficult to ignore what goes on in the body and not to focus on it, but it does seem to be what I see and feel. I wish to perceive you and focus on you instead. I cry out to you in my weakness. I am grateful for having energy to complete tasks, food to eat, loving people in my life, sleeping well and so much more. I am most grateful for the hope you have given me. Help me out of this bodily "winter" into a bodily and spiritual spring. Grant me your mercy. Grant me your peace. Amen.

January 28
The Lord led me to re-read one of my books, *YOU CAN HEAL YOUR LIFE* by Louise Hay.[1] Oh, my gosh! I realize that I have been harboring a resentment toward another person for the past 3 or 4 months who had gotten too close to me and begun to meddle in my personal affairs.

I had to send positive thoughts and prayers to this person, imagine the best for the person, and send them love and grace. I said aloud, "I forgive you for X (I named what they did) and I forgive you for Y (I named what else they had done.)" I had to really mean it (which was difficult).

At first, my condition (sinus, cough, etc.) got worse and then it began to improve. It is truly a law of nature that how we think and feel shows up in our state of health. I read it so many times, but forgot about it in this instance. I asked God for help and now know why I couldn't accept peace and healing. Once I discovered my underlying issue and accepted the peace and sent it to another, I improved. Thank you, Lord.

January 30
I finally decided to go to the doctor since I still have some symptoms hanging on. I went to a clinic and got a very

young doctor who asked what I was doing to treat them. I said that I was doing nasal washes, taking oregano pills, an herbal sinus relief medicine, and Echinacea. I expected him to roll his eyes, denounce it all, and write me a prescription for an antibiotic. Surprise!

Instead, he commended me for what I was doing and stated that when natural means are used, the body has an amazing capacity to heal itself. After examining my nose and such, he said that I looked pretty good and to just continue what I was doing! And he said I didn't need an antibiotic! I couldn't believe it! He confirmed what I had hoped—that natural methods were working. I had also purchased a product called Cedar X™, an herbal aromatherapy formula developed locally, which helped tremendously with the cedar pollen. Thanks be to you, Lord!

February 6
Hallelujah! The sinus infection is completely gone, the cough almost gone, and the laryngitis almost gone! I am so happy to be doing better! I still have to see the person with whom I had been upset. Now, even though I see them often, things are better and I just forgive them if they do something that tries to irritate me.

Beyond the Senses

We live in the world. We see with our eyes, hear sounds, taste food, feel with our skin, have nerve endings on the skin for every organ in our body, smell good food cooking, and yet, there is much beyond what we perceive. Therefore, when any illness manifests itself, we tend to concentrate on what we are experiencing. I had been doing that for the past two months. The lesson I learned from this was two fold. The first part is to do a mental and spiritual check of how we are feeling every day. If we are disturbed by a chronic situation and we are not at peace, it will eventually affect us in some way if it is not resolved. In my case, my resentment may have contributed to the development of the symptoms or at the very least, exacerbated them. It was right in front of my face, yet I did not see the problem.

We get so caught up in our own personal dramas and emotions that we are unable to step back and see where it is leading. I was literally experiencing the "congestion" of my own resentment and ill feelings. I was blocking the Lord from healing me or acting through me. Have you ever added chocolate syrup to milk? Do you notice that even just one drop begins to change its total appearance? What about one drop of resentment in the bottle of the milk of health? Or one drop of fear? Or one drop of anger?

Forgiveness is another attribute to the kingdom. It is time to forgive ourselves and others. Maybe we harbor something from long ago in the past. I thought I had forgiven positively everyone, until a person mentioned someone that we both knew. I immediately went into the attack mode and said some unflattering things about the person of whom we were speaking. Later, reflecting upon my day, I knew that I needed to forgive and to forget. How do you know in your heart if you have forgiven someone from the past or who has recently hurt you? You will know because you no longer have the desire to speak ill of them or to tell others how much they hurt you by what they did or said. For many people, ex-spouses fall into that category. If it is a current irritation in your life, steps must be taken or prayers said to resolve it or it will eat you up from the inside out, which delays your own healing.

My friend Maggie had tiffs with different members of her family in which they would go months without speaking, usually over something very trivial such as who would have Easter dinner at their house. She felt that they should give her a break because she had cancer. Let's face reality here. After the initial shock is over and one has been undergoing cancer treatment for some time, all breaks one gets from sympathy are over, and it's back to whatever the relationships were before. I was surprised when one of the organizations I belonged to gave me an "unexcused absence" from a meeting, when I was too weak to attend the meeting from undergoing chemotherapy, and didn't call and say I wasn't coming! We cannot count on "the sympathy factor" to resolve long or short standing conflicts or to change circumstances. It is best to take steps to resolve them ourselves.

The second part I learned was that if we perceive ourselves to have an illness or condition, it is quite a challenge to get beyond what we are currently experiencing and, instead, to concentrate on the spiritual and physical wholeness inside ourselves. If a person is not healing, it is time to ask the Lord to reveal what the real underlying spiritual or emotional problem is. In addition, ask the Lord to lead you to anything you might need nutritionally. Ask Him to help you "see" yourself or another person as well and happy. With people praying for you right at this moment, ask God to let those prayers well up inside of you like a spring and flush out the darkness so it can be replaced with light. Do not live by the five senses. Pray to go above and beyond them into the realm of total health. This requires great faith on your part—faith to believe in what you cannot yet see. Faith will be discussed more in depth in a later chapter.

February 7
Lord, I hope that I am truly healed of EVERYTHING. Help me to see what I cannot see, to know that all is well. I guess I should get a CAT scan someday.

"All I see in you is perfection, wholeness, and beauty. You have part of me and thus, my own beauty is present. You are beautiful." O, Lord, I thank you for your goodness and kindness. I certainly haven't felt beautiful, especially lately. I know that beauty is a heavenly attribute. There is the beauty of what is seen and the beauty of what is unseen. Thank you for "scanning me" down to the core of my spirit and seeing what I need to see in myself. If only others could realize how beautiful they are to you, things would be so different. Unfortunately, we often listen to other voices that aren't so kind over the years and we accept society's definition of beauty. Thank you for letting me know that you alone see what is beautiful in a soul. I blush with joy at your reminder of who I am. May I reflect your beauty unto the world. Amen.

Inner Wholeness and Beauty

Many of us have childhood memories or teenage memories related to our sense of "beauty" as it relates to ourselves. I remember when I was young, my mother had five of us to contend with, so she didn't want to spend long hours fixing our hair. To this end, she gave my sister and me "perms" which made our hair very kinky and fuzzy. Even now, when I look at my grade school photos, I cringe. We always walked to school and when we got older, our school chums would drive by in their cars and yell out the window, "Hey, banana nose!" My sister and I ran home and told our dad that someone called us "banana nose" like Jimmy Durante, the famous comedian who had a gigantic nose! I became very self conscious about my nose even though I tried not to be. I dated someone later on who offered to pay for a "nose job" if I wanted one! How do we feel beautiful amidst that kind of abuse? My dad even tried to tell us to be proud of our nose because it was indicative of our Italian (Sicilian) heritage. *You are fairer than the sons of men...The king's daughter is all glorious within. (Psalm 45:2,13)*

When we become ill in any way, we get even more self-conscious of how we look because we know people are making comments about it when they see us. Lately, I had felt pretty ugly with a red nose and watery eyes. What a sight that was! When I was losing my hair due to chemotherapy, I definitely did not feel beautiful. But, I lost sight of what "beautiful" really meant.

I am thinking of an old "Twilight Zone" show on television from years ago. I have never forgotten it because it impacted me greatly. The entire episode revolved around a woman who was in a hospital bed with her faced wrapped entirely in bandages. The doctors and nurses were gathered around her bed talking about the surgery and whether or not it was successful to fix her face and make her "beautiful" like the rest of them. I waited on edge as they got ready for the moment of revelation and slowly began to unwrap the bandages. When her face was totally revealed the doctors and nurses all gasped in horror because the operation had been unsuccessful. But the camera hadn't shown her face. How bad could she possibly look? I sat on the edge of my chair saying, "Come on! Show us her face!" With great sadness they handed her a mirror and she, too, was horrified and disappointed at how she still looked. Finally, the camera showed her face—and it was absolutely beautiful! Then, the camera showed the faces of the horrified doctors and nurses and they had the most ugly pig-like faces. What a surprise ending, but it sure made a strong point. We can't always trust society's definition of beauty.

Just think about it for a moment. Haven't you seen some animal or insect that God created and thought to yourself, "Boy, God, you sure did create one ugly beast!"? That is merely your interpretation of what you have seen. They are all beautiful to the Lord. Surely, we top all other creatures in beauty to Him, because we are made in His image. I remember when I went to the first meeting at the holistic clinic and there were musicians there who sang a song that stated, "How could anyone ever tell you, you are anything less than beautiful?" Michele, the director, looked me directly in the eye as she sang these words walking among the guests, and I just began to cry.

Why am I even mentioning beauty? I wondered that myself. After receiving the words from the Lord, I know that not feeling beautiful is another hindrance to healing. When one doesn't feel beautiful, one is not at peace. It takes peace to heal. Be at peace and know that we are all beautiful to the Lord who created us. *You are altogether beautiful, my darling, and there is no blemish in you. (Song of Solomon 4:7)*

Heavenly Pearls of Wisdom

Move beyond what you see and feel. What you are feeling and seeing is not the real you. Ask God to reveal obstacles to your complete health.

Forgive and resolve conflict. Even small issues can block the healing process. Being free of these allows healing to flow through you.

You are beautiful. See yourself as God sees you—a beautiful part of Himself that he has created. Radiate that beauty.

12
God's Mission Revealed

February 18

"Take time to listen to my counsel. Man speaks much but listens little. There is much I could reveal if man would only listen. He has closed his ears to my voice. And, at times, when man does hear me, he refuses to believe that it is me. He believes that it is his own conscience. I am his conscience and so much more. I am the brain, the heart, the liver, the hands, and the feet. I am every part—spiritual and physical. Recognize me. I am here—like a child waiting patiently for his playmate.

Oh, the joys we could experience together! That is why I created you--for us to be joyous together! My joy is completely fulfilled in my creation. My joy is to be shared. Joy is an emotion that you can feel. You are always asking to 'feel' my presence. Every time you feel joy, you are feeling me. Find, in your day, moments in which you find delight. I share that delight with you. Then, spread that joy to others. This is a gift to give others that is more precious than gold—the gift of joy—the gift of me. Amen."

Finding Joy

No matter what condition the body appears to be in, there is some moment in which we find delight—an unexpected phone call from someone we care about, something inspiring that we read, a kind word someone says to us, a small favor that is done for us. Mother Teresa talks much about joy and its value in the spirit world. She said, "Jesus is the love to be loved. Jesus is the joy to be shared. Jesus is the peace to be given."[1] At any time, when you feel even an instant of joy or gladness, you are feeling the presence of the Lord. For He is joy and gladness personified. We have festival grounds directly behind our home. One weekend, I walked outside to feed the birds and heard the most beautiful Scottish music, including bagpipes! My heart instantly felt uplifted. Apparently, a festival called "The Highland Games" is located there every year. For me, there is just something about Scottish music and bagpipes that tug at the heart strings. I just love both Scottish and Irish music. That was a moment of joy for me and I could hear the band at no cost.

The Bible also speaks constantly of joy. *You will make known to me the path of life; your presence is fullness of joy; In your right hand there are pleasures forever. (Psalm 16:11)* This is another truth revealed, one we don't often think about. Joy IS the presence of God. We sometimes forget the joyful moments because they get overshadowed by anything negative that doesn't make us feel good emotionally. Every day, there are moments and instances of joy. Grab hold of those moments, delight in them, and thank the Lord for letting you "feel" His presence!

Not everything joyful that happens in the spiritual kingdom is approached with loud bells ringing, shouting, or trumpets blaring. Some moments of joy are quiet and personalized for your heart only. Let your heart make a joyful noise to the Lord. *Make me to hear joy and gladness... (Psalm 51:8)* In other words, "Don't let me forget what small moments of joy are, Lord. Remind me that they are evidence that you are right here with us every moment." *They who dwell in the ends of the earth stand in awe of your signs; you make the dawn and the sunset shout for joy. (Psalm 65:8)*

February 22
Today, I shall make it totally a day of thanksgiving to the Lord for all of his abundance—no asking for anything (that will be tough for me). I seem to spend one minute in thanksgiving and the rest of my prayer time asking for much. Not today! Today is totally praise, gratitude, joy, and excitement at being one with the Lord. I simply wish to bask in His presence. *God mounts the throne amid shouts of joy, the Lord amid trumpet blasts. Sing praises to God, sing praise, sing praise to our King, sing praise. (Psalm* 47:6-7)

February 23
Miguel, another acquaintance from our real estate office, has been diagnosed with stomach and liver cancer. He has been throwing up and has lost over 40 pounds. At first, he thought it was just acid reflux and so did the doctors. They kept giving him different medicines for bleeding ulcers and finally tested him. He called me today for advice and I am overwhelmed. Where do I start? How do I systematically arrange all twenty things that I have been doing, so that someone who is scared and has been given a serious diagnosis knows where to begin? Oh, help me Lord, but also, help him and have mercy on Miguel. O, Lord, I just can't stand by and let another "innocent" die from the poison of chemotherapy if they prescribe it. I must let him know that he has other options. I need your guidance, Lord. I humbly ask in the name of Jesus. Amen.

February 24
The doctor told Miguel that he is terminal. I told him, "Miguel, do NOT accept that for one minute! He doesn't know a thing about you. Do not believe it or you will internalize it and then you will make it happen." He starts chemotherapy in a few days and I don't want him to take it. I know what it will do to him—it will kill him. I know it in my very

being. If he is supposedly "terminal", then WHY are they giving him chemotherapy? Help us, O Lord. I am asking you for the truth that only you can give. I pray for Miguel because he is so afraid. What can I do through you, Lord? For it is not I, but you that work in me. Amen.

February 24
Today is a beautiful sunny day! I called Miguel and he was unable to get his first dose of chemotherapy. Because he has been bleeding from the stomach, his red cell counts and hemoglobin were too low. He's already in a bad state. I'm afraid that if he takes chemotherapy, it will cause a rapid decline. I told him about the holistic clinic and about all the books that I have read. I know that he feels overburdened, because I too, have been in that saddened, bewildered state of confusion. I encouraged him to at least call the clinic for information. O, Lord, help him to find whatever will help him live. Amen.

February 27
I visited Miguel at his home today and took him a book. It is strange but somehow, I feel God calling me on this "mission" to help another person and to be the true friend I want to be to another. I hope that Miguel reads the book soon. He needs to start making drastic dietary changes TODAY!

I read in the book, *THE SEVEN STOREY MOUNTAIN* what Thomas Merton so aptly stated. People would ask him what he wanted to be while he was in college and one of his friends revealed to him that his answer should be, "I want to be a saint." If we desire it, God will help us achieve it.[2] So, I want to be a saint. There are no ifs, ands, or buts. What a tough "career" that is! Mother Teresa states, in a book of her writings called *MOTHER TERESA, NO GREATER LOVE,* that the first step to becoming holy is to will it. She also says that holiness is the greatest gift that God can give us because it is for that reason that he created us.[3] I will it, Lord. Amen.

March 1
Thank you, God, for another month! I talk to my mom and dad every week on Sunday night and I miss them dearly, being several states away in Iowa.

Lloyd and I visited Miguel together today. I can't believe this—I asked him why the doctor is having him take chemotherapy. He said it was to make Miguel more comfortable! What kind of crock is that? It is going to make him feel like hell, that's what it will do. He's already throwing up and this will make it worse. His blood counts are down and chemo will only make those worse. What is the doctor thinking? Is it just because he doesn't know anything else? Is it to help cancer treatment centers stay open? Is it because of the influence of the drug companies? Is it to protect the doctor from lawsuits for not providing "standard of care"? (I'm really beginning to detest that term.) Is it the money to be made from chemotherapy? Lord, reveal the truth to me! What is the sense? Am I missing something? How did we get in this predicament? Oh, answer me, Lord, when I am listening. Amen.

"As man turned away from me and my spiritual laws, he embraced what he calls 'science'. Science encompasses only my physical laws and the physical laws became man's new 'god'. The first commandment has been violated over and over. In always searching for 'scientific proof', other gods have been put before me. *I, the Lord, am your God...you shall not have other gods besides me. (Exodus 20:2-3)* **And mankind is reaping the rewards of another 'god'. And the reward is his own death and destruction by the scientific 'creation' of harmful compounds that should never be used in the body that I created for man in my wisdom and benevolence.**

What you call the laws of nature are really the combining of my spiritual and physical laws. These are man and I co-existing. The fact that my sun shines on your body, warms the skin, letting it manufacture vitamins, is such an example. These are the laws that I created for your health and well be-

ing. No matter how much man tries, he cannot manufacture the sun or the moon. 'Scientists' have removed me (the true life source) from the picture and left only the corpse (death and destruction). *Your perversity is as though the potter were taken to be the clay: As though what is made should say of its maker 'He made me not!' Or the vessel should say of the potter, 'He does not understand'.(Isaiah 29:16)* **Pray for My return to man's consciousness of all processes, all life, and all nature. I am not in an atomic bomb, a bullet, nor any type of harmful chemical treatment. These are not in conjunction with me. I am in clean air, life giving water and food, sunshine, herbs, and all things living. Find me once again and healing of body, mind, and spirit shall follow. Tell man to find me. I am here waiting patiently while I watch many of my people being destroyed. Seek me and find me and return to my laws of nature—the way I set them up from the beginning. Amen."** *God makes the earth yield healing herbs, which the prudent man should not neglect."(Sirach 38:4)*

March 5

I spoke with Miguel's wife yesterday after his first chemotherapy. He vomited all morning the next day and slept the rest of the day. O, Lord, I turn him over to you. **"I will take care of him, Diana."** Does that mean that you will heal him? **"That is between Miguel and me."** But, he wants to be healed. **"Only I know his inner being."** But, Lord, I want him to be healed! **"What you desire for others, they must choose and claim for themselves when their state of being allows such a choice. He must choose for himself."** So, is there any more I can do for him as a friend? **"Continue to offer help as I direct you and pray as you have been doing."** I will tell him that he must choose life and claim your healing grace. I do claim your mercy on us all. **"My mercy I give freely. Teach him of my mercy. There are lessons to learn."** May I continue to learn them, too, O Lord. **"Indeed, I love a willing heart and a faithful student."** Blessed be your name forever. Amen.

March 7
Miguel called last night. He is weak but he wants to go see the herbalist! Also, he sent in his deposit to the holistic clinic. I am so happy for him. He has chosen life, I believe. He goes for chemo again in three weeks. Oh, I wish he would quit chemotherapy. Lord, direct us both. I humbly bow before you.

March 11
I took Miguel to see the herbalist and after much talk and questioning, we left with a sack full of herbs and tinctures. Already, Miguel's stomach bleeding has stopped. Hallelujah! But, he is severely anemic and has lost 45 pounds. O Lord, I send him light and healing. I think I'll also mention the foot pads I'm using. He needs every possible thing to give him a leg up on this. O Lord, is there anything I need to know?

"Know that I am well pleased with you, my daughter. You have laid down your life for another. It does not necessarily mean that one must cease to live on earth. One can lay down one's life by setting aside time for another, praying for another, consoling another, or doing a good deed for another.

For in these moments, your life is suspended as I (through you) enter into their life. This is pleasing to me. In that moment, you become my minister, my healer in whom I am well pleased. I have answered your request from the heart to be a better friend—now you know. A true friend expects nothing in return and you are that friend. I was a friend to my apostles and I loved them dearly. One may have many acquaintances but very few friends. Cherish the ones you have and the ones who have you as a friend will cherish you. Amen." *There are friends who destroy each other, but a real friend sticks closer than a brother. (Proverbs 18:24)*

Detoxifying from the Outside

I mentioned liver detoxification, which occurs from the inside out. However, we can additionally detoxify through the skin. The skin is the largest organ in the body and many of us do not think of it as an organ like the heart or liver, but it is. It contains three layers and through pores, has a very unique system for absorbing and releasing. It also contains glands such as sweat glands. One of the best ways to detoxify the body through the skin is to sweat. When we sweat, there is much more in that sweat than meets the eye. Sweat normally contains many chemicals including sodium chloride, urea (a waste product of metabolism), and 2 and 4 methyl phenol. Additionally, it can contain any substance that is overloading the body in its attempt to eliminate the excess.

I first noticed how powerful this is by accident. When I was in my early 30's, I had surgery to remove my uterus because it had prolapsed (fallen). When I returned home, I quickly became fatigued each day for weeks. Somehow, I felt that my body was "hanging on" to the anesthetic that they used in surgery, but I had no clue about how to get rid of it. One summer day, I decided to just get outside in the sunshine and watch my husband do some outdoor work. The summer days in Texas get very hot, usually around 95-100 degrees. Therefore, it didn't take long, sitting outside in the heat of the afternoon, to break out into a sweat. Soon, I was sweating profusely, but it seemed to feel good. (Usually I can't stand sweating like that when I'm not doing anything athletic.) After about an hour, I finally went in the house and took a shower.

I couldn't believe it. The next day I woke up and I had more energy than I'd had in weeks! I actually felt pretty good! It's funny how sometimes you just know something, even though you didn't read it anywhere and no one told you. I just <u>knew</u> that the intense sweating had removed the remnants of the anesthetic that were in all of my tissues. Later, when I heard about ways to detoxify through the skin, I was already a believer in how powerful that could be. A few weeks ago, I called Angie, one of my clients. She had painted the living room, had all of the windows open, the air conditioner turned off, and was shampooing her rugs, in the middle of summer. I said, "You must be sweating profusely in there! It's 102° outside!" She laughed and responded, "I prefer to think of it as detoxifying!"

I learned about three choices that one could use to help with external detoxification and I'm sure there are many more. From the clinic, I used a substance called Liquid Needles™ (which can be ordered through the internet) and added 4 ounces of this body soak to a hot bath in which I would soak for 20 minutes. This company makes several types and the one I used was labeled CAN-133 (standing for cancer). Later, I used two other types of detoxifying soaks. One was Dr. Singha's Mustard Bath™ and the other was Liquid Needle™ Lympha soak, which is designed to clear the lymph nodes. When the body begins to remove toxins from the blood, they are carried by the lymphatic system to the lymph nodes. Sometimes, the lymph nodes get backed up and need to be 'cleared'. The body soak may aid this process.

Another product that Angela introduced me to was detoxifying foot pads. I was very skeptical at first, but decided that I was going to avail myself of every possible natural avenue to return to health by giving them a try. They are sold under various names, but all work essentially the same. They are not cheap, but at the very least, they are fun to use. Right before going to bed, a pad with detoxifying agents is placed on the bottom of the foot, in the area of the arch. A type of medical tape is then applied to hold the pad in place. As we sleep, the pad draws out harmful substances through the skin of the feet. The foot pad will turn brown or green as it soaks up the substances. People argued that they could pour water on the foot pad and get the same result. However, one can pour water on a t-shirt and it will look the same as a t-shirt that someone has worn and sweated in, but they are definitely not the same. You cannot see the chemicals and harmful substances being eliminated with the naked eye.

I will say this about the pads. For the first time in awhile after I started using them, I slept like a baby! That alone was worth it to me and if they were removing harmful substances in the meantime, more power to them. I love those things! I wanted many types of ammunition in my arsenal. This was just another one. I found the foot pads at the local drug store and some grocery stores. They can also be purchased online. I have fun with those!

The final external and internal detoxifying method I use is massage therapy. In the beginning, I read that it was helpful in the healing process but didn't understand why. Upon further reading, it seems that massage is important for the nerves in the body, as well as the obvious muscular relief. In Tanya Pierce's book, *OUTSMART YOUR CANCER: ALTERNATIVE NON-TOXIC TREATMENTS THAT WORK*, she talks about the protocol advanced by Dr. William Donald Kelley. He gave five essential parts of treatment that are imperative for healing from any type of illness. They are: 1) Nutritional and enzyme supplements, 2) detoxification of the body, 3) nutritional diet, 4) neurological stimulation, and 5) spirituality.[4] Some of the benefits of massage are that it can enhance immunity by increasing the flow of lymph, increase circulation to certain areas, improve the quality of sleep, relieve pain, and relieve anxiety. And the best part is that all of the "side effects" are good ones! Massages used to be considered unnecessary pampering. Now, many people realize the many and varied benefits of these effective practices.

Craniosacral therapy (CST) is a form of light touch that involves the brain and spinal chord and the balances and rhythm between them. CST was started by Dr. William Sutherland in the 1930's and is gaining in popularity for relief from a variety of ailments.[5] I had that done twice and liked it. It felt very warming and comforting to my body.

There are many wellness spas and clinics that offer these services or if one asks friends, the name of a good massage therapist usually comes up in short order. We are only one or two people away from finding any person that we wish to find.

March 12
I am now aware of God's mission for me at this point in time. My current mission is to be a true and good friend to Miguel. It seems to me that God gives us mini-missions and when he places it in our heart, we are so happy to do His bidding. When we complete that mission, he places another, bigger one in our path, but gives us the tools to complete it. I think many times we worry about what our mission is and quite often it's really a set of mini-missions all strung together, with some more challenging than others. We help others and we grow spiritually in the process.

In the political arena, the government has given many banks and auto makers money. They have dubbed it a "stimulus package". Well, in assigning us our mini-missions, God gives us our spiritual stimulus package. It is called "grace". Thanks for your "spiritual stimulus package", Lord! Your grace is always such a blessing and I wait for your next "assignment".

March 14
We found out today that one of Lloyd's acquaintances, Angelo, died of stomach cancer at age 44. He took the full rounds of chemotherapy and only lived 8 months after the diagnosis. O, Lord, this is getting ridiculous—thousands of dollars of treatment to live a few months and die a slow painful death? He would have lived almost that long without treatment. The clinic also lost a patient. He had come with liver cancer. He had finished the full course of traditional treatment, waited quite a while, and then decided to go the holistic route. The staff there said that he waited too long. Bless them both and all of those who can't afford to do holistic treatment because insurance doesn't pay for it and bless all of those who don't know that another choice exists.

I dreamed I was working in a scrap metal yard. Is the scrap metal yard those people who are poor in spirit and need my help? Or are they the people who have been "thrown away" by conventional medical treatment? Lord, only you can answer that. What will the next mission be? I will work wherever you send me. I am yours and not my own. Amen.

Heavenly Pearls of Wisdom

Grab the moments of gladness. Joy is "proof" of God's presence.

Be there for others. It is part of your mission from God.

Detoxify on the outside too. Get your fill of massages, baths, and foot pads. They are not just for "pampering" but for healing.

13
Living in Faith

March 15, later in the day

"Take the faith I give you and place it in your heart so that it may grow. Use the faith—faith without works is dead. Go about every small task with faith—faith in my love for you, faith that all is well, faith of your fathers before you, faith to act, faith not to act but to pray. Only then can the world be healed, through those who are faithful (full of faith).

Those who do not have faith run to the wrong source for help and guidance. *O faithless and perverse generation, how long will I be with you? How long will I endure you? (Matthew 17:17)* **I am the only source. It is faith that moves mountains—it is faith that will change the condition for which you cry out to me. If one did not have an ounce of faith, one would not cry out to me at all, but seek other sources first. Then, when those failed, they would possibly remember to cry out to me. Only faith can save you. It is my spiritual law and it is a powerful one.** *I say to you, if you have faith the size of a mustard seed, you will say to this mountain, 'move from here to there' and it will move. Nothing will be impossible for you. (Matthew 17:20)*

Man abides by the physical laws that he can see, but does not abide by the spiritual laws which he cannot see. That

is why faith is another key to the kingdom. It is a paradox. One must have faith to 'see' the spiritual laws in effect and yet faith IS a spiritual law unto itself. Faith is not something one can see in action, yet it is there. Faith conquers much evil. Pray for faith."

Faith Saves Us

I mentioned faith briefly in another chapter, but after the Lord's message, it needed even more attention. Faith is another one of those small words we hear that has a magnitude of meaning. Some forms of faith are so simple because we see certain things demonstrated over and over so we have faith that they will occur. For example, when we pick up the telephone, punch in a number, and hit "dial", we have faith that it will do exactly that every time. Or if we hit "talk", we have faith that there will be a dial tone there. I call this "easy faith".

But what about the "hard faith"? It is so much harder to believe in something we don't see with our eyes, can't smell, can't hear, or can't taste. When we've never experienced something before, how are we supposed to have faith that it will happen? The Bible contains countless examples of the faith that people exhibited, often in the face of ridicule. I am thinking about the sinful woman who came into a home where Jesus had been invited. She came up to Jesus weeping, washed his feet with her tears, wiped them dry with her hair, put perfume on them and kissed them. Jesus did not say, "Well, you are pretty good-looking, so I think I'll forgive you today." Nor did he say, "You are a great foot washer, so you are forgiven." What he did say was that her sins were forgiven. And he followed it up with, *Your faith has saved you; go in peace. (Luke 7:50)* Faith saves us!

Faith also heals us. There was a woman who saw Jesus in a crowd. She had female problems with bleeding for 12 years. She came up behind him and touched the outer garment he wore. *She said to herself, 'If only I touch his cloak, I will be healed.' Jesus turned and saw her. 'Take heart, daughter,' he said. 'Your faith has healed you.' And the woman was healed from that moment. (Matthew 9:21-22)* Jesus didn't say He healed her. He said her FAITH healed her. That just amazes me. My faith in Him can heal me?

I still must be reminded of this lesson often when I become weak or frustrated with situations or start to worry about my health. Faith means that we are "confident" in the Lord's power. As the Lord told me, faith is a gift. We can't "work at it" like we are used to doing when we are trying to achieve something. No matter how much I squeeze my eyes shut and say "I have faith!" I cannot make it happen. I can repeat it over and over and not see or feel any change. It is a GIFT. You cannot earn or work at a gift. *For it is by grace that you have been saved, through faith—and this not from yourselves, it is the gift of God—not by works, so no one can boast. (Ephesians 2:8-9)*

Faith seems to be on a type of continuum. One can have no faith, a little faith, some faith, weak faith, strong faith, and so on. And it varies from situation to situation. We may have a strong faith in one situation and a weak faith in a different situation. A Canaanite woman approached Jesus and begged him for mercy for her daughter who was possessed by a demon. They had a verbal exchange in which she persisted. *Then Jesus answered, 'Woman, you have great faith! Your request is granted.' And her daughter was healed from that very hour. (Matthew 15:28)* I noticed that he didn't say, "You have an itsy bitsy bit of faith." Therefore, it seems to me that in order to experience what our heart desires, we must have a whole lot of faith—in fact, great faith! But, to Jesus, you need only have faith the size of a mustard seed. Have you ever seen a mustard seed? They make necklaces with a mustard seed in them. I bought one to be reminded of this fact and the seed itself is not very big. It's round like a peppercorn and approximately 1/20th of an inch.

So, we are back to the question, what can we say or do when we are on the low end of the faith continuum in a situation? Yes, you are getting it and I hope I am getting it too. We can pray for the gift of faith to be given to us. We can and should pray for faith when it is lacking, especially when it comes to healing. God is already leading you where you need to go and in what you need to do. We must pray to accept the gift of faith. It seems weird, but we cannot "see" the good that is being manifested if we have no faith and we can't achieve faith.

We have to ask God for faith and he will not refuse us. He will not. He is all goodness. It is not in His nature to be mean. It is his nature to be kind, good, and loving. And He gives freely of His mercy and faith. Remember the prayer from the words of scripture that we discussed before. "I believe, Lord. Help me in my unbelief." And then I add to that, "Grant me the gift of faith, for in this situation I am weak. Grant me the confidence to trust in you. Let me, too, be saved by faith." *And the prayer offered in faith will make the sick person well; the Lord will raise him up. (James 5:15)* The faith must come first in order to offer a prayer in faith. Pray to recognize when you don't have enough faith. Pray for faith in each situation. *Is any one of you in trouble? He should pray. (James 5:13*) When He gives you the gift of faith, hold it in your heart and pray for faith in the next situation. We will know when we are truly "in Him," when we have great faith, no matter what situation presents itself to us. *I am glad I can have complete confidence in you. (II Corinthians 7:16)*

March 16

Today I went to the health club and saw a girl name Fay. She told me that her forty-year-old brother had died of stomach cancer. She said one of her sisters-in-law had ovarian cancer, had surgery, took chemo, and had surgery again. This all sounded like what the doctor wanted to do to me. She is now taking MORE chemotherapy and is in absolute pain and misery. Good grief! Fay asked what I would recommend. O, my God! Where would I start? It's already so late in the game. They have already poisoned her beyond belief, overwhelmed her liver, and caused more tumors. I gave her a couple of suggestions, but my heart wasn't in it because I was too discouraged and heartbroken. I went on to yoga class.

My heart was so heavy with the sadness and senselessness of it all that during class I began to cry and pray. O, God, once again I cry out to you! Help these people! Keep the medical profession from killing more people with poison that only works in a very few instances! More innocents are dying! It's worse than World War II with the number of deaths. Help us! I don't know what to do! I am so overwhelmed! I want to help them, Lord. Where is my faith now? My faith shatters constantly and must be rebuilt by you. I heard these words, **"Diana, do not take on this burden. It is too much for you to bear. Give the burden to me. I am the Lord of all—the guilty and the innocent. Just as in your World War II, it took much time and many deaths before people rose up, as groups, and said 'enough'. When enough people have died from 'the cure', a revolt will slowly begin to occur. People will come out of the darkness and see the light of truth. Like the evil marching armies in World War II, this evil can also be stopped.**

Insurance companies will begin to see the fallacy in current treatments, will refuse to pay the high cost of them anymore, and will force physicians and other medical and scientific personnel to find better, more natural, effective ways of dealing with diseases of all kinds. Methods previously shunned will be accepted and the light will come forth. As you have seen, you received natural treatments at your holistic clinic for over one year at less than half of the cost of just one of the poisonous treatments. It will start with the insurance companies. In the beginning, the motive will be to save money. Money will still be the concern rather than actual health and well being, but good shall come forth from it. Remember, give the burden to me and I will begin to harden hearts that need to be hardened and soften hearts that need to be softened. It has begun. Amen."

Give me courage and faith, Lord, to hold on and to believe that these changes are coming. Right now, it seems so hopeless, just like it did to the people in the prisoner of war camps.

Share the Burden

No matter what you or a loved one is going through in your life, the burden is not yours alone. In fact, maybe it shouldn't be your burden at all. The Lord had to tell me not to take on certain burdens. They are simply too much. Scripture speaks often of burdens and what to do or not do with them. There are examples in which people were overwhelmed just as you or a loved one has felt, just like I feel at times as I continue to heal. *I cannot carry all these people by myself; the burden is too heavy for me. (Numbers 11:14)*

I had cried out to God for all of the people who are suffering with cancer and getting chemotherapy or other treatments that are harmful to them. That prayer was immediately heard and I must now have faith that the Lord is already manifesting in others a desire to remove or lighten the burden that I feel. I want to help so badly and yet feel helpless. Maybe you feel helpless for yourself or another. *I will come down and speak with you there, and I will take of the Spirit that is on you, and put the Spirit on them. They will help you carry the burden of the people, so that you will not have to carry it alone. (Numbers 11:17)*

Give the burden to God. It sounds trite and is an easy thing to say, but it is very difficult for us to do. When I am carrying something that is too heavy or awkward and someone says, "Here, let me carry that for you," I am so relieved because I can walk easier or get where I am going faster. That person usually walks with me until I arrive at the point where they can deliver the item they are carrying. I do not worry that they will drop it or give it back and say, "Forget it! This is too heavy!" I have placed my trust in that person to carry the item I treasure safely to my car, home, or other destination. It is much more difficult to do that on the spiritual plane. We say we give the burden to God and then we struggle with Him to take it back. *Praise be to our Lord, to God our Savior, who daily bears our burdens. (Psalm 68:19)* Wow! We can give Him our burdens EVERY day. We just have to remember to do it.

Sometimes, giving the burden to God is merely telling Him that it is too much for us to bear. Jesus himself said, *Come to me all you who are weary and burdened, and I will give you rest.* (Matthew 11:28) It is not your responsibility to heal others or yourself. If you will it and give the burden to the Lord, he will show you what needs to be done and effect the changes in you that are necessary. That is where the faith comes in once again. That faith part is pretty darned important.

> March 17
> I had a dream last night that I was somewhere near downtown and had my arms full of items I had purchased. It was dark and the stores were closed. Fearfully, I headed toward my car. When I got to the parking lot my car was gone! The dream then flashed ahead and I was at a charity affair. They had discovered who had taken my car, but apparently I did not take it back. I had been driven to the charity event by a chauffeur!
>
> This dream had much meaning. A car represents our life. If we are driving, we feel in control. If someone else is driving (such as a relative or friend), then we feel that they are controlling our life. Aha! The symbolism here is that my life is not my own—once I gave up my car (my life) to a higher power, I received something even better (the chauffeur driven car) in return. God took the car! And along with the car (my life), He took on the burden of all of the maintenance and upkeep! Thank you Lord! What awesome ways in which God chooses to teach me.

Life-Giving Water

Let's take a brief look at the type of water we are drinking. Does it make a difference? Yes, it does. In this world we live in, our livers already have to contend with so many toxins in everything, including water. Water that comes into your tap is clean by your city standards, but it is still full of things for which your city does not test. Think about all of the things running off into your water supply. There are pesticides, herbicides, chemicals from the pipes themselves, and more items than I could possibly mention here. My parents live in an area where the river water is run through a plant, cleaned, and sent out as tap water. Some places use recycled sewer water. Water can contain any runoff from factories that "dump" waste into the rivers and metabolic waste from all of the drugs we take. One town found that the drinking water contained high levels of the excreted form of anti-depressant drugs because so many people in the town were taking them. *The fish in the Nile will die, and the river will stink; the Egyptians will not be able to drink its water. (Exodus 7:18)*

What is the answer then? To be 100% sure of the water you drink, it is best to drink steam distilled water. Distillation raises the temperature of water until it becomes a vapor. At this temperature and pressure, the chemicals and toxins will settle out of the vapor, the pure vapor collected, and the vapor cooled to become water again, minus all of the impurities and harmful toxins. *He draws up the drops of water, which distill as rain to the streams; the clouds pour down their moisture, and abundant showers fall on mankind. (Job 36:27-28)* Man used to catch rain water and use it for everything. Unfortunately, we cannot rely on what the distilled water vapor picks up from our atmosphere anymore. With all of the unseen pollutants in the air, rain water is often full of sulfuric acid or any other number of compounds. So, we've actually sort of returned to the old days in which people used to boil their water to make sure that it was safe to use, but steam distillation is a better process. *Worship the Lord your God, and his blessing will be upon your food and water. I will take away sickness from among you. (Exodus 23:25)*

I think it is interesting that God spoke about blessing the food and water in the sentence right before removing the sickness. Do you think there is a connection? Absolutely. Water helps carry away toxins and waste that produce sickness. How much should you drink? It is best to drink approximately 60 ounces daily. How much is that? Most household drinking glasses today are 12 ounce glasses. They used to be 8 ounces, until we began, through the decades to super size everything from drink to food portions. 'Supersizing' water portions is a good thing. Most of us don't get enough water, especially those who choose to drink coffee, tea, or other caffeinated drinks. Therefore, one would need at least 5 twelve ounce glasses of water a day. I drink a 12 ounce glass as soon as I get up in the morning, then I have a 12 ounce glass with breakfast, lunch, and dinner, and finally, a 12 ounce glass in the evening (not too close to bedtime!). Do coffee, tea, and colas count as water? I heard a doctor counter this question with this. Would you wash your hair in tea or coffee or cola instead of water? The obvious answer is no. She then followed up with, "Then, why would you bathe your kidneys and tissues in coffee, tea, or cola? Do you honestly think that will help the cells in your body get rid of waste material?" Not only that, but I would not want to drink a type of water that may remove some waste from my body and then deposit something else in my tissues. I rest my case, counselor.

Steam distilled drinking water is available in most grocery stores. We have the five gallon drums delivered here to our home and use a water cooler. The water tastes so much better. I remember that, where I grew up, the water in certain areas tasted like iron. Ugh! We use the distilled water for cooking and making coffee or tea. Your kidneys will love this type of water and so will your liver.

Why not drink spring water? We could, but is the source of the spring water still trustworthy? I saw an article recently in the newspaper which stated that cement plants emit thousands of pounds of mercury into the air every year. Where does all of that mercury end up? Does it end up in those natural springs? Research would be in order to determine how companies that sell water test the water quality.

Does the "natural water" truly come from the mountains or some other uninhabited region? In many countries, trash is dumped in the mountains. The water will still contain any minerals or non-usable chemicals it picks up as it flows downstream. The kidneys then have to work to eliminate the unusable minerals. Distilled water gives the kidneys a much-needed break and allows them to more efficiently excrete waste from the tissues. Spring water would be preferable to tap water in some instances, but I believe that distilled water is still the best bet. *I will lead them to brooks of water, on a level road, so that none shall stumble. (Jeremiah 31:9)*

March 24

Lately, I've been praying for several people, mostly members of my own family. But I begin to wonder—is this really doing any good? Lord, is the spiritual realm as powerful as we think it is? How do I know I am even helping anyone? **"Diana, the purpose of my coming to earth was to help people know my Father, but also to overcome the world—to demonstrate that the spirit world (My Father) is the ONLY power. My dying and rising was so much more than just a victory over death. It was to reveal the ONE and ONLY power—not evil, which had presented itself as a power, not fear, not greed, not kings—NOTHING of the earth world which is visible. The invisible is all in all. Faith is the key to the invisible—my purpose was to restore faith in my Father and His promises.**

When one has had an internal wound that is stitched and the outer skin stitched over it, one can no longer see the wound. But, due to the manifestation of my being in every

cell, one has faith that the wound is indeed healing, even though it is invisible to the eye. My earthly mind had to have faith that my Father was going to work all good through me. You and others must have faith that when you pray for anything or anyone with a humble and sincere heart, that spirit receives that prayer, becomes part of that prayer, and is changed. If your heart is humble and not self-righteous, your spirit grows in grace also—again not visible with the human eyes. Pray always—as often as you are able." *By faith, in the name of Jesus, this man whom you see and know was made strong. It is Jesus' name and the faith that comes through him that has given this complete healing to him, as you can all see. (Acts 3:16)*

Heavenly Pearls of Wisdom

We must have faith. It heals us. Rely on faith. If you don't have it, pray for it.

Give the burden to heaven. It is too much for you on your own. The Lord will help you.

Drink distilled water. It is pure and has no chemicals or metals in it.

Let God Take the Car. Ask God and let Him guide you. He is the vine. You are the branch. The branch does not worry in which direction it should go.

14
Renewal of Spirit

Importance of Sleep

The importance of good deep uninterrupted sleep cannot be overemphasized for overall health, but also for healing of body, mind, and spirit. We have heard stories of how prisoners of war were (and probably still are) tortured by depriving them of sleep. Horrible changes occur in the body when it cannot have time to rest and renew itself as God intended. *I will lie down and sleep in peace, for you alone, O Lord, make me dwell in safety. (Psalm 4:8)* Sleep brings different brain rhythms, allows the subconscious to work out problems encountered in the daytime, allows the immune system to remain strong, the body to repair itself, and so much more.

Half of America is sleep deprived. We do too much and we rest too little. It seems to be the expectation. There are numerous articles proclaiming this. Looking back, from a personal standpoint, I realize that I used to be extremely tired. Some of it was sleep deprivation. When I worked a full time 8 to 5 schedule, I was rising at approximately 5:30 am and going to bed at approximately 10:30 pm—sometimes later. That equates to about 7 hours of sleep or less. I know for a fact that my body needs at least 8 hours of sleep and often, 8 and one half hours. Therefore, at the end of the work week, I was already five to six hours short. I attempted to make it up on weekends, but we all know that weekends are the main times we have to catch up on yard work, laundry, cleaning, errands, run children to and from lessons, etc. Where does the time go?

I was attending school at night to get my doctoral degree, which was a 3-hour drive one way, and I usually fell asleep halfway through class. I would "study" at home on weekends and fall asleep. I just couldn't catch up. I thought this was how it is in the work world. You work hard, get tired, work more, get more tired, and receive a paycheck. Period. Even Jesus must have been fatigued. How could anyone sleep through a storm on a small boat, for Heaven's sake? *Then he got into the boat and his disciples followed him. Without warning a furious storm came up on the lake, so that the waves swept over the boat. But Jesus was sleeping. The disciples went and woke him saying, 'Lord, save us! We are going to drown!' (Matthew 8:23-25)* Although the lesson is not about how tired Jesus was, can you imagine how exhausted he must have been to still be asleep when waves were crashing over the boat? I'm fairly certain that my knees would be quaking and I'd be wide awake.

Later, I took a job in which I traveled from 60-200 miles per day to visit different small towns. I vividly remember driving down a highway heading to a small town and falling asleep at the wheel. I pulled off of the road and took a 10 minute nap in order to continue. When I was at the office, I would put my head down and fall asleep at my desk. Sometimes I thought the workday would never end. I went to the doctor because I was fatigued constantly and he said rather flippantly that as long as I wasn't falling asleep in the middle of eating, I just needed more sleep. He told me not to worry about it. A few years later, blood work revealed that I had contracted the Epstein Barr Virus, which brings on great fatigue that flares up off and on.

My last 8 to 5 position was as a school administrator and by this time, the tiredness and fatigue were unbelievable. I thought it was just stress, but I fell asleep on the bed in the evening when I arrived home and was changing out of my work clothes. "If I can just lie here a moment, I'll feel better," I told myself. To my surprise, I would wake up at 9 or 10 pm and it was almost time for bed! And I still needed supper. What was wrong with me? I fell asleep in trainings or would fight my eyes rolling back into my head during meetings. If I called in sick because of a migraine headache and to catch up on sleep, I had double the phone calls and work waiting for me when I returned. Does this sound like the hamster in the little cage running and running and sleeping in a cage? At least he gets his full amount of sleep. *I have labored and toiled and often gone without sleep... (2 Corinthians 11:27)*

The point I am trying to make here is that the need for sleep and what it means to the body cannot be ignored without a price to pay. People will brag about how LITTLE sleep they need. Don't listen to this. Everyone's body is different. You will know how much you need when your body is allowed to fall into its natural sleep pattern. For many of us, this is usually only possible during vacation, when people are allowed at least two weeks off to go to bed at night when we want to and get up in the morning without an alarm clock!

If you are getting plenty of sleep and still feeling tired, something is amiss. It is imperative to get to the source of this tiredness. It is not normal. Do not make excuses. You should have plenty of energy throughout the day.

Many people have trouble sleeping. My husband is sometimes one of those. We personally do not take any prescriptions for this because they have undesirable side effects, as with any prescription, because it is an isolated chemical compound. Of course, we know not to drink large glasses of water or drink alcohol before bedtime, but we still might need a little help sleeping through the night. Sometimes, off and on, he will take an herbal supplement or product to maintain a deep sleep. One he likes is called Dreamboost®. Some people drink Chamomile tea, others take melatonin. Find what works for you if you need something like this. We do not take anything for an extended period because the body gets used to it and the effectiveness becomes diminished or non-existent. For me, taking a yoga class makes me sleep better than a baby and one of my friends said the same thing. There must be something to it.

March 27
While meditating and reading my Bible, I came across these words: *...unless you turn and become like children, you will not enter the kingdom of heaven. Whoever humbles himself like this child is the greatest in the kingdom of heaven. (Matthew 18:3-4)* O, Lord, I humble myself at your feet. I imagine you sitting on a rock and myself sitting in the grass with my head in your lap, trusting, being held, carrying on a conversation, and being taught. Many times, I feel like a child—so dependent on you and so loved by you. Continue to teach me and hold my hand as I walk my story.

"I am here holding your hand and when two people walk holding hands, they move as one. Move with me and I move you forward toward great rewards. As I walk with you, we join hands with others on the path and continue to move as one. So it is with my kingdom. We all move and live and have our being with the Father as one. Take the spiritual hand of all you meet. If they will not take your 'hand', then move on to the next one. That is how changes are made—by unifying in spirit. When hearts are unified by spirit, much change occurs and the kingdom rejoices just as it does when one lost soul returns. Take my hand and let us walk together." Lord, I humbly take your hand. Where you lead, I follow. Do not let go of my hand, for I am a child and do not wish to stumble. Amen.

Remain Humble

Humbleness is often confused with humiliation. This makes people afraid to be humble. Being humble in our society is associated with being a servant, weak, being trod upon, a wimp, made fun of, given lesser jobs, or making little to no money. What we often fail to realize is that some of the greatest and most well known people retain a sense of humbleness. Humbleness means giving credit to others, not always having to seize the limelight, a desire to help others without being constantly recognized for doing so, being content not to sit at the head table, and so on. The Bible speaks often of humbleness and humility for those are the traits of the kingdom.

Pride often gets in the way of total healing. We are proud of the way we look, the family we are born into, the success we have, the type of career we have, the degree we possess, the mind we have, the possessions we collect, the home we live in, or the neighborhood. There are countless ways in which mankind has "false pride." Pride makes us stubborn. In order to heal, we must recognize that the only pride we are allowed to have is the pride that comes from being in Christ. Anything else is fantasy which leads to misery. One of the hardest lessons I learned was to be humble; to me, humility was demeaning. Now I know that humility brings freedom. Freedom brings joy and excitement. Joy and excitement bring healing. *When pride comes, then comes disgrace, but with humility comes wisdom. (Proverbs 11:2)*

We can lose everything in an instant, including our health and vitality. I can't really analyze the degree of pride that I might have had before this all happened. *Before his downfall a man's heart is proud, but humility comes before honor. (Proverbs 18:12)* I can only say that I have been extremely humbled by it all because it made me fully aware of the fact that without God we are nothing. Humility brings the wisdom to understand and to rejoice in it.

Humility makes us want to do good things for other people, even if we don't reap any immediate rewards. *Who is wise and understanding among you? Let him show it by his good life, by deeds done in the humility that comes with wisdom. (James 3:13)* God wants us to take the hand he offers us, but not with pride and high-five slapping. Instead, we take his hand with head bowed in reverence and a gentle slipping of our hand into his, as little children.

What do we do if we don't know how to be humble? Or what if we don't know if we are humble? We pray and ask the Lord to show us where we are not humble and we ask him HOW to be humble. He will let us know in the stillness of our hearts. Do you know people who will anonymously do something kind for another? That is a sign of humility. Recently, I saw some Girl Scouts® selling their trademark cookies outside of a local store. I went up to the table and let them tell me about all of the kinds of cookies. Then, I got my wallet out, extracted the money and gave them enough money for two boxes of cookies. But, I told them that I did not want the cookies. I instructed them that the next person who bought cookies was to be given two free boxes as a bonus. They looked at me somewhat mystified, but agreed to the terms. I left the parking lot smiling to myself because of how fun that had been. No one would know who to thank, the girls sold two boxes of cookies, and some lucky person would get extra cookies for the freezer or to give away. And I would put on no weight!

The following week, the church had a raffle and folks were outside selling raffle tickets. I heard one couple saying that they wished they could buy a ticket. So, I asked Lloyd for the money (since I don't carry my purse to church), walked up and gave them the money for a ticket. I said, "I want to donate to the raffle, but I don't really want a motorcycle. Will you buy the ticket and keep it so I can make a donation?" They smiled hesitantly and said they could do that for me. Another fun deed. *Humble yourselves, therefore, under God's mighty hand, that he may lift you up in due time. (I Peter 5:6)*

Have you seen someone lead a project and then give lots of credit to all of those who worked with him/her? We've all seen people who like to steal the credit, but to see the opposite is most refreshing. Let us be the ones to give others credit before ourselves. There is great healing in all acts of humbleness. A pilot, Captain

Chesley Sullenberger nicknamed "Sully," landed a passenger jet in the Hudson River when it was evident that it would crash. He successfully set the plane on the water, which enabled all of the passengers and crew to be rescued before it sank completely. Afterward, there were many award ceremonies in his honor. However, at each and every one, he said that he was only doing his job and that the true thanks went to the River authorities and those who had rescued the plane passengers. He remained humble. *For everyone who exalts himself will be humbled, and he who humbles himself will be exalted. (Luke 14:11)*

March 31
Monday was supposed to be Miguel's first appointment at the holistic clinic but he had to go to the hospital! His blood count dropped too low, he got very weak, and he couldn't keep food down. Oh, I wish he would not have taken the second chemotherapy treatment. But he has to discover his own path. He should be out of the hospital soon.

I finally got up the nerve to go to the laboratory and have my blood drawn for blood chemistry and a CA-125 for cancer and guess what? That lab no longer does the CA-125! Now, I have to go to a doctor and get him to order it for me. What a bother. And I was <u>finally</u> mentally ready. I'm going to pray about who to call—Lead me Lord. Good night.

April 3
The church had a service for the Stations of the Cross, which Lloyd and I participated in. After we made our presentation, I heard these words, **"My daughter, I am well pleased. Because you have answered my call and obeyed me, I have bigger things planned for you. Remain humbly in my service and look to me for all. I love you because you are my own and only desire what is best for you, to share in my happiness and love."** Lord, I do humbly wish to serve you in good health and peace of the Spirit. Amen.

April 7
I saw Miguel at the clinic meeting last night. He has started going to the clinic, but plans on taking the next chemo treatment. I am disappointed in that but he believes that it is the right thing to do and I must respect his decision. Since the 2nd treatment landed him in the hospital, I hate to think what the 3rd chemo treatment is going to do to him. I've got to stop thinking this way and think success for him. But, I am seeing more and more people die from the treatment.

Tomorrow, I am going to see my primary care physician and ask him to order my CA-125 since the independent lab I go to no longer does them. Lord, why must I go see him? **"It is not for you. It is for him."** For the doctor? **"Yes—it is I who use you for my work—it is not about you."** But, Lord, it sure seems like it's about me since I am the one living this. **"Remember, Diana, it is about ME, demonstrating My glory and truth. Do not question where I send you."** O, Lord, help me—give me courage. I rely on you alone to fulfill your promise and I humbly serve and obey you. Amen.

I Sent a Prayer

Today, I sent a prayer written on a scroll to Heaven.
It flew attached to the wings of a dove.
The dove returned to me with a scrolled message.
It said, "You are mine and I love you."
I sent another prayer written on a scroll to Heaven.
It flew attached to the wings of a dove.
Jesus appeared in front of me holding the dove in His hand.
He gave the dove to me and said,
"My peace I leave you."
I held out my arms to hug Him, so grateful was I.
He stepped forward, I thought, to hug me.
But, he stepped <u>into</u> me instead.
I felt only love as I stood holding the dove.
Not I, but he that liveth in me.
He stepped into me and we became one.

April 10
If only I can hold on to that feeling of oneness. Thank you, Lord, for the beautiful experience. I could not have dreamed that up if I tried. Today is Good Friday. I stand at the foot of your cross, ashamed at what we have done, and continue to do, to you. You agreed to this punishment on the cross for our sake and I am deeply grateful. You were hidden from our view for a few days while God worked great changes in you through the darkness. Work changes in us through our dark times, too. I love you Jesus. Amen.

April 11
I went to see my primary doctor. I did receive the blood work for only the cell counts and all is well except my white count which is still only 2.3. The doctor gave me lab orders for a CA-125 and a CEA, which I'd never heard of. Apparently, it tests for cancer in the abdominal organs. He also ordered a white and red blood count. I plan on having a normal count and normal markers the next time around. Lord, let me see my wholeness through you.

April 12
Christ is risen! Hallelujah! I had a wonderful day with family. God bless us all as you always do. Amen.

April 13
My friend from the office, Grace, is going to work at the clinic part time! Good for her! She was diagnosed with breast cancer, took no chemotherapy, only went to the clinic and is now doing absolutely great!

I saw Miguel again this evening. He is doing better and gets the next chemotherapy treatment tomorrow. I pray for him.

April 14
I haven't sold any homes so far this year, my slowest year yet, but I know the Lord will bring them to me when the time is

right. All is in Divine right order. Sometimes, it is hard not to feel inadequate by human measures of success. I know that all human success quickly fades away but Spiritual success is of His kingdom. Lord, I bow humbly before you in my sense of inadequacy, for only you can make me whole—how do we feel whole?

"It is I that fills in the gaps of human weaknesses. It is I that makes you whole. You are incomplete without me. Do not be tempted to look at everything through the eyes of inadequacy. Look through my eyes. See what I see. I see each person as a manifestation of me—nothing less. If you fall prey to seeing only as man sees, you will never find peace and happiness for man will always see to it that you fall short. Man is a terrible assessor of other men. That is best left to me. *But when they measure themselves by one another and compare themselves with one another, they are without understanding. (2 Corinthians 10:12)*

You may not judge yourself either, for you have not yet gained wisdom. Pray for wisdom. You are at the crossroads and wisdom will guide you. But, you must ask for it as another gift of the Holy Spirit. Then, wisdom shall go forth before you to discern situations and to judge motives. You are never permitted to judge the heart of another. That is for me alone.

A heart that turns to me is never judged harshly, but is judged righteously. Turn to my tender heart. I cannot say that enough. *And if anyone hears my words and does not observe them, I do not condemn him, for I did not come to condemn the world, but to save the world. (John 12:47)* **Turn to my heart, receive the light, and walk out in it. Remember, I am the one who fills the gaps—I make you whole. See, all things are new Amen."**

Lord, I ask you big time to help me feel and act whole, grant me the wisdom I need for every need, every situation, every solution. Know, my God, that I thank you for not judging me harshly. I turn my heart humbly to you. *Fear not, I am with you; be not dismayed; I am your God. I will strengthen you, and help you and uphold you with my right hand of justice. (Isaiah 41:10)*

Wisdom Guides Us

When I was in the early stages of healing, I wasn't able to focus on the concept of wisdom. I was concerned with staying alive in the physical realm. Now, two years later, I see with clarity the importance and necessity of the spiritual gift of wisdom. Wisdom allows us to "know" how to think, how to pray. Wisdom dictates what we need to do or not do, who we need to talk to and who we need to avoid.

There are entire passages in the Bible devoted to wisdom and yet, for the longest time, the concept of wisdom was just a word to me—an unobtainable trait. *Whatever wisdom may be, it is far off and most profound—who can discover it? (Ecclesiastes 7:24)* Wisdom seemed reserved to only certain people like Solomon, the Dalai Lama, the Pope, or people who have lived a long time here on earth (with, of course, God being wisdom Himself). *God gave Solomon wisdom and very great insight, and a breadth of understanding, as measureless as the sand on the seashore. (I Kings 4:29)* How could ordinary individuals be granted wisdom?

I suppose all of us possess some degree of wisdom. It is a never-ending scale and multifaceted. Some of us are wise in certain circumstances and challenged in others. What we hope for is to make advances along the continuum. I definitely need to pray every day for wisdom and understanding. *Who endowed the heart with wisdom, or gave understanding to the mind? (Job 38:36)* It is a spiritual gift, just like the gifts of peace and faith.

It is a gift that cannot be "forced." We can't line up a check list of things to do or accomplish to obtain wisdom. *For the Lord gives wisdom, and from his mouth come knowledge and understanding. (Proverbs 2:6)* It is a gift that comes to us as we encounter each new or repeated situation and pray. It is granted to us to the measure by which we can comprehend and absorb it. Even Jesus had to tell his apostles that he couldn't tell them everything because it was too much for them to "wrap their head around" (as my daughter Angela says). *I have many more things to say to you but you cannot bear them now. But when He, the Spirit of truth, comes, He will guide you into all the truth... (John 16:12-13)*

I purchased some religious books several years ago in my quest to become holy and "enlightened." Most of those books ended up gathering dust on the bookshelf, unfinished. They were "too heavy" for me to comprehend at the time. One such book I remember is titled, *Crossing the Threshold of Hope* by Pope John Paul II.[1] He said, upon being interviewed about how and why to pray, "We begin to pray, believing that it is our own initiative that compels us to do so. Instead, we learn that it is always God's initiative within us..." No way! That concept went way over my head at that time and now it makes perfect sense to me. The Lord will grant us each wisdom as we pray for and need it. *If any of you lacks wisdom, he should ask God, who gives generously to all without finding fault, and it will be given to him. (James 1:5)*

Have you ever encountered a child or person of whom others are in awe? They say that he or she is "wise beyond their years." Apparently, these young ones are receptive and ready for God's wisdom. I remember when I was about 10, one of my friends, Charmin, who visited her grandmother next door, wanted to become a Christian. My memory is somewhat foggy, but she asked me to baptize her. We had no river, nor pond, not even a swimming pool nearby, but I agreed. The best I could do was to turn on the outside faucet and get as much of her under it as possible. (I'm glad our parents didn't find us or they would have thought I was trying to drown her.) I believe this was God's wisdom and guidance already at work in me and in my friend too. People marveled at the wisdom of Jesus, because, at a young age, His wisdom surpassed the wisdom that had been demonstrated by any previous or current generation. *"Where did this man get these things?" they asked. "What's this wisdom that has been given him, that he even does miracles? Isn't this the carpenter?" (Mark 6:3)*

The earthly world does not tend to operate on "wisdom." Attaining wisdom does bring some sorrow, because the wiser we become, the more we come to recognize that the world operates on greed, jealousy, fun for the moment, television, careers, and electronics. *For the wisdom of this world is foolishness in his sight. (I Corinthians 3:19)* Where and when is the opportunity for spiritual wisdom to be granted?

If I had possessed the wisdom I have now, would I have done anything differently? Maybe. Would I have prayed differently and thought differently? Most assuredly. Wisdom guides us to truth. Knowledge and internalization of that truth re-creates how we pray, how we think, act, and re-act or don't re-act. Once we have wisdom we move and act more in unison with the Lord within us. Everything changes. We impart that wisdom to others. *But the wisdom that comes from heaven is first of all pure: then peace-loving, considerate, submissive, full of mercy and good fruit, impartial and sincere. (James 3:17)* We become that wisdom.

In a book entitled, *THINGS VISIBLE AND INVISIBLE,* author Guiliana Cavallini talks of the images used by Catherine of Siena, a well-known Catholic saint. She was considered one of the great doctors of the church. Her thoughts and reflections (dictated to others) made connections between the simple tasks of her very ordinary life at home with her parents, and the magnificence of God. She likens us to a log that is thrown on the fire. At first, the log resists the flames and just seems to sit there. Eventually however,the fire singes that outer bark and begins to burn through the log, igniting it, moving toward the center. And finally, as the fire roars, the log and flame are one—the log becomes the flame.[2] Remember, you are becoming the flame—Him. Pray every day for wisdom and it shall go before you. *I keep asking that the God of our Lord Jesus Christ, the glorious father, may give you the Spirit of wisdom and revelation, so that you may know him better. (Ephesians 1:17)*

Heavenly Pearls of Wisdom

Get the sleep you need. Find a way. Your health is at stake, your driving safety, and your emotional well being.

Find humbleness. Let go of pride. Then, healing and wisdom will follow.

Pray for Wisdom. Accept it as a gift in all parts of your life and it shall guide you, rather than fear.

15
The Flower Blooms

Cottage Cheese and Flaxseed Oil

Every week, my intent was to give Miguel a new, natural, anti-cancer, health-promoting piece of information. This week, I felt that he was now ready for a simple mixture to add to his diet. I called him.

"Hi Miguel! How are you feeling today?"

"Hello, Diana! I am very tired, but I am able to keep my food down and that makes me happy."

"Miguel, you feel tired because the chemotherapy continues to destroy your red blood cells. The tired part is hard to compensate for. I'm glad you stopped taking those awful prescription iron pills. How is the liquid natural vegetable iron working for you?"

"It is much better for me because the prescription iron pills made me so constipated that I was most uncomfortable."

"Well, I have something new for you to try this week! We want to press in on all sides to get you well. Do you ever eat cottage cheese?"

"No, what is cottage cheese?"

"You don't know what cottage cheese is?" (One, I could tell that he'd never had to go on a diet and two, it never dawned on me that a person from Latin America would not have eaten cottage cheese!)

"No, I don't. Tell me, please."

"This will sound horrible, but it really does taste ok. It is a form of curdled milk." There was a slight pause.

"I am not familiar with that. Why are you asking me about this cheese?"

"I want you to take 1/4 cup of cottage cheese and mix it in a blender or with a hand mixer with one tablespoon of cold-pressed flaxseed oil that contains lignans (like Barleans™). Cottage cheese and flaxseed oil, which has Omega-3 and Omega-6 fatty acids, work together to make those oils very absorbable by the cells of the body. You can also add a little apple juice to make it more pourable."

"Because I am not familiar with this cottage cheese, can I use yogurt?"

"Yes, you can use yogurt with no sugar, but you will need ¾ cup of yogurt to one tablespoon of flaxseed oil. From what I read, the doctor that discovered this, Dr. Johanna Budwig, used a substance in her native Germany called Quark, but we don't have that here so we use cottage cheese. Cottage cheese and yogurt contain sulfur based protein. When these combine with flaxseed oil, the body can now use it to carry oxygen to the cells by producing hemoglobin."

"Ok, I will give it a try. I want to do what I can."

"Good for you, Miguel. I'll talk to you in the next few days." (I really wanted him to stop the chemotherapy, but he was too afraid. Fear is a terrible thing when dealing with disease.)

"Ok, Diana—Ciao!" (Apparently, they say ciao in Latin America just like we do in Italy—what a surprise!)

Lloyd was standing nearby as I talked on the phone. He asked me further questions.

"Diana, I couldn't help but overhear and I have some questions about this Budwig discovery. Exactly how is eating cottage cheese and flaxseed oil related to cancer?"

"Well, Dr. Budwig discovered that people with cancer were missing phosphotase and lipoproteins in their blood. Plus, they had some sort of greenish substance in their blood serum that other people did not have. She then figured out that these things were related to a deficiency in essential fatty acids—primarily Omega 3 and Omega 6."

"Why are Omegas so important for the body?

"They help carry oxygen from the membrane to the center of the cells for respiration. They also help build new cell membranes for use during cell division, and they produce substances which help the immune system."

"But how does this relate to cancer?"

"When cells don't get enough oxygen due to faulty membranes, they eventually convert to using sugar and becoming anaerobic cells—the famous cancer cells."

"I'm beginning to understand."

"Do you know that cells need the lipoproteins to build the cell membranes that hold the cells together? And if there aren't enough lipoproteins present when the cell is ready to reproduce, a "faulty" reproduction occurs—again leading to cancer cells that contain twice the number of chromosomes."

"Why don't we get enough essential fatty acids, like Omega 3 and 6?"

"One reason is that natural plant oils, that have been removed from the plant by man, have been run through a chemical process called "hydrogenation," to increase shelf life and keep them from going rancid. (I think they call them trans fats.) We ingest these oils in salad dressings, margarine, fried foods, and other condiments."

"And why is that so bad?"

"Because the body cannot use these altered fats. It rejects most of them and they end up clogging arteries, veins, and organs. Some altered fats are taken up by the body because it thinks they are cholesterol. This causes the cell membranes to be altered in such a manner that they cannot produce hemoglobin to carry oxygen to the center of the cell. They are missing the electron cloud necessary for oxygen to be attracted to them—again setting the stage for formation of cancer cells."

"And this can be helped without harmful drugs?"

"Yes—by mixing the two simple ingredients of cottage cheese and flaxseed oil."

"What changes occur in cancer patients when they get Omega 3 and 6?"

"Dr. Budwig observed that in just 3 months, people with cancer returned to normal levels of phosphotases and lipoproteins and tumors started to disappear."

"How long do people need to continue eating cottage cheese and flax oil?"

"Dr. Budwig recommended continuing for 3 to 5 years, even though most people had marked improvement in just a few months."

"Why aren't more people doing this?"

"Lloyd, you know it's just like everything else we studied. Someone suppresses the information. In this case, her own boss at the institute for which she worked had patented the hydrogenation process. He didn't want this information to get out because it contradicted his work. So, she got fired and couldn't get anyone to publish her work due to opposition from the huge margarine industry which relies on these oils."

"You're right. I should have guessed it would be something like that. So often, it's about money, the bottom line for most people. Anyway, now I see why you keep putting cottage cheese on the store list."

"And all this time you thought I was watching my waist!"

"Diana, it sure beats the hell out of what I saw you go through with chemotherapy and it's a lot cheaper too!"

"D'accordo!" (Italian for "I agree"!)

April 15 (Tax Day!)
When we attended Michele's meeting at the Holistic Clinic on Monday, she said something that resonated in me. She stated, "There is a solution for everything." We must pray in every situation for the solution and let grace flow through us. If the channel is blocked, we cannot receive when the solution comes. Meditating on this is very profound. The scripture is full of examples of amazing solutions that God provided for his people in distress. Here are just a couple of them.

Moses parting the Red Sea is a great example of an extraordinary solution to a most pressing dilemma. For years, the Israelites had been slaves of the Egyptians. After some convincing by God, they set the Israelites free. They immediately regretted it and decided to recapture them and bring them back after they had already left Egypt. Moses answered the people, *"Do not be afraid. Stand firm and you will see the deliverance the Lord will bring you today....The Lord will fight for you; you need only to be still." (Exodus 14:13-14)* When it seemed hopeless because the Egyptians were about to overtake the Israelites, the people cried out to God and the solution was provided! *Then the Lord said to Moses, 'Why are you crying out to me?'...Raise your staff and stretch out your hand over the sea to divide the water... (Exodus14:15-16)* The Red Sea parted and the people walked across on dry land to the other side. When the Egyptians followed them, the sea swallowed them up. Who would have thought of that solution?

Jonah getting spit out by the whale that had swallowed him was another solution. Jesus multiplying five loaves and two fishes to feed thousands was another dynamic solution. These are ALL solutions! A miracle, then, is simply God's solution! God works FOR us!

O, God, thank you for solutions. We just ask and every need is supplied. We may not always know what the solution will be—many times it is more wondrous than we can imagine. You are awesome, Lord!

"I am willing to grant so much to my people. They must turn to me for everything. Remember, I am the way—the way to what? I am the way to the solution. Someday, you will learn that I am the solution. That is the true union with me. Amen."

April 18
This morning, I went outside to feed the birds and discovered that one of the birdfeeders had been knocked to the ground and the lid removed by a raccoon. As I approached, I saw a dove stuck inside of the tubular-shaped structure! It could not turn around, could not back out of it, for the fit was too tight. It opened its wings as much as it could in the confined space, and fluttered frantically, especially when I picked up the feeder with the dove inside.

I tried shaking the feeder upside down hoping the dove would fall out. It didn't work and it just got more flustered. I tried to reach my fingers in and hold its wings down, but I could only get one wing and then it would flap the other wing furiously. I took a deep breath, calmed myself down and talked to the bird.

I said, "You know, if you found a way in, we can figure a way out, but you must remain calm for me so that I can help you." After a few more unsuccessful attempts, the bird finally became calm and stopped fighting me. I was able to grab both wings, fold them around its warm little body, and pull it out backwards. The second I got him out, he plopped onto the ground and flew off immediately! Yippee! I was jubilant that he had escaped unharmed.

Later, in reflecting upon the incident, I knew it was symbolic in meaning. Many times, we experience a situation from which we cannot extricate ourselves on our own. But we think we can. We struggle and try and try with all of our might and will. It doesn't work. When we find calmness and relax and remember to ask God for help, He takes over. It might be uncomfortable as he presses in our wings, but he is working to set us free from the "prison" of the situation. What an analogy!

Lord, help us out of our "tight spaces" that we get ourselves into and even those that aren't our fault. Help us when we can't help ourselves. Help us to find calmness and to ask for your help—to wait patiently for it. For you will free us from what binds us and you will rejoice when we "fly"! Amen.

There is Always a Solution

I came across a beautiful paragraph by Thomas Merton that states,

> *"He (God) was surrounding me constantly with the work of His love, His wisdom, and His mercy. And so it would be, day after day, year after year. Sometimes I would be preoccupied with problems that seemed to be difficult and seemed to be great, and yet when it was all over the answers that I worked out did not seem to matter much anyway, because all the while, beyond my range of vision and comprehension, God had silently and imperceptibly worked the whole thing out for me, and had presented me with the solution. To say it better, He had worked the solution into the very tissue of my own life and substance and existence by the wise incomprehensible weaving of His Providence."*[1]

While you are speaking, God is already answering. We are just like the dove stuck in the birdfeeder. It is best to stop struggling to find the answer, calm down, and ASK God to take the burden. He is already taking it AS you ask! What a difficult concept to comprehend but that follows the law of the spirit world of God! Unfortunately, that is what caused Jesus to say that if the person thought lustful thoughts about another, that they had ALREADY committed a sin in their heart. The thought already did it for them! We can use this in a positive manner and believe with all of our hearts that our cry to God is a thought that is already being acted upon for our good! *Before they call, I will answer; while they are still speaking, I will hear. (Isaiah 65:24)* There are many instances in the Bible in which things occur WHILE someone is still speaking! Here are just a couple of them. *While Peter was still speaking these words, the Holy Spirit came on all who heard the message. (Acts 10:44) Peter said to Jesus, "Lord, it is good for us to be here. If you wish, I will put up three shelters—one for you, one for Moses and one for Elijah." While he was still speaking, a bright cloud enveloped them, and a voice from the cloud said, "This is my Son, whom I love; with him I am well pleased. Listen to him! (Matthew 17:4-5)* (Of course, I'm sure it was quite unsettling for the apostles to see Jesus speaking to two people who had been dead a very long time!) The point is that while you are busy speaking, God is already doing something related to the situation.

This brings us back to the trust and belief issue again. All one need do is ASK, trust that God is already answering, and believe that something is going to change. It always does. We live in a world where NOTHING stays the same—ever. Let that fact work to our advantage when we are ill or having a relationship problem or financial troubles. It WILL begin to change as soon as we ASK the Lord for help. Is it going to change without His help and guidance? Yes. Will it be the same help as if we had asked? Maybe. Will we ourselves change and grow after we have asked? Yes! Will we grow and change if we don't ask for His help? Probably not, and that is why we may be doomed to relive the situation again or another one just like it. We are here on earth to "get it." We are to learn truths and to become Him.

Every day in my diary, I wrote key words at the top of the page. For many days, my key words were ASK, TRUST, BELIEVE, RELAX, and RECEIVE. When that dove was stuck, I kept repeating "There is a solution, there is a solution."

While I was speaking and praying, confessing my sin and the sin of my people Israel, and making my request to the LORD my God for his holy hill, while I was still in prayer, Gabriel, the man I had seen in the earlier vision, came to me in swift flight about the time of the evening sacrifice. He instructed me and said to me, "Daniel, I have now come to give you insight and understanding. As soon as you began to pray, an answer was given, which I have come to tell you, for you are highly esteemed. (Daniel 9:21-23)

This passage tells me that we don't always recognize the answer when it comes and sometimes, the Lord has to "send" someone to help us with the insight and understanding to recognize the answer or the solution. The Bible doesn't use the word solution, but God's answer IS the solution.

I'd never touched a dove before in my life. Once I calmed myself down and quit trying to shake the poor dove to pieces, the answer came. Reaching my fingers into that tube and holding the dove's wings closed became as natural as drinking my morning beverage, just not quite as relaxing!

Sometimes, I witness another possibility. People present God with their problem, and then when God sends an answer, they reject it. I see it happen when people ask me for information in the natural healing realm for themselves or a loved one and then refuse to consider those options because it is "too much work" or because someone else told them not to do it. If they prayed on it, God brought them to new knowledge as the answer, and they refused it, what then? I cannot tell you the consequences of this because only God himself knows. Someone I know prayed for a good job. A great job interview came along promising good pay, they went to the interview, and then told the interviewer that if they were to get hired, they needed a higher salary than was advertised because it was a 45-minute drive from their home to work and it was going to cost them too much in gas! (I probably don't need to tell you the outcome of this interview.) I think wisdom says that when God sends the answer, take it! If we aren't sure if the answer or solution is from God, what do we do? We ASK Him to reveal whether it is from Him or not. We pray. He will answer.

April 23
I called Miguel and he is in the hospital again! I am amazed that he answers his phone no matter where he is! But, this pains me. He took the 3rd chemo dose and apparently, his liver tumor shrunk, BUT his stomach tumor GREW! They put two stints into his intestines, one from the stomach to the small intestine to allow food to pass through, and another one somewhere else. He is going to continue taking chemo but the doctor is going to switch to a different chemo drug. I am disappointed that Miguel is going to stop going to the holistic clinic because he is afraid that the colonic treatment will interfere with his stints. I am beginning to lose hope for him. He is acting out of fear. We usually don't make good decisions when that is the basis of our choice. O, Heavenly Father, hear my prayer for him. He walks in darkness. Let him be guided by you and not by fear. Help us all, Lord, to trust in you. Help him to see the light. *...he who walks in darkness does not know where he is going, while you have the light, believe in the light that you might become sons of light. (John 12:35-36)*

April 30
I saw a greeting card today that someone had sent me and it said something like, "Remember, every flower that bloomed had to go through a lot of dirt first!" I definitely have experienced all types of "dirt" in my life. I have experienced the quicksand of financial troubles, the rocky soil of troubled relationships, the shifting sand of life in general, the desert of loneliness, the swampy part of betrayal, and the depleted soil of sickness.

Lord, please help us all through our times "in the dirt," for sometimes, we feel that we are sinking and the dirt is about to fill our nostrils and choke us.

"I reach with my right hand and pull you up. You must reach up with your hand in the certainty that I will grab your

hand and extricate you from your circumstances. After I pull you up slowly and have set you gently upon the rock, then it is I who lifts you up to new heights, allowing your feet to leave the ground.

In the time of darkness, I am working changes in you or any of my children experiencing the darkness. My sons Abraham and Moses had their periods of darkness also, but I used that darkness to bring about great leaders. My son, Jesus, allowed darkness to completely swallow him. Then, he was lifted up for all to see for the glory of My name.

Tell my children to extend their hand in prayer to me. I <u>will</u> pull them up out of their darkness, whatever it may be, so that they can experience my light. They need the rock to stand on and I <u>am</u> that rock. I provide all if they look to me—abundance, money, a companion, a gentle loving heart to share, health, and spiritual strength. Rely on Me. The seed grows so slowly and I make the way through the "dirt." The plant grows stronger day by day, the bud appears, and yet growth is still occurring. *Your people shall be just, they shall possess the land. They, the bud of my planting, my handiwork to show my glory. (Isaiah 60:21)*

Then, from one day to the next, the blossom appears in all splendor—the beautiful manifestation of me is demonstrated to the world, to do the work I have set before it, to give me glory. Amen." *Consider the lilies, how they grow: they neither toil nor spin; and yet I say to you, even Solomon in all his glory was not arrayed like one of these. If then God, so clothes the grass, which today is field and tomorrow is thrown into the oven, how much more will he clothe you...?(Luke 12:27-28)*

May 7

I called Miguel again today to check on him since I didn't see him at the meeting. He was not able to receive his next chemo dose because his blood counts were too low. He is very, very tired and I am not able to help him. He is continuing with juicing and enemas and so forth which seem to help him. His weight goes down right after chemo and then he is able to bring it back again even though he is still grossly underweight. His doctor seems surprised that he is doing this well, acknowledged that Miguel was doing other holistic things, and encouraged him to "keep it up." Too bad the doctor himself can't look into these things for fear of being labeled a "quack" or being ostracized by the medical community.

Lord, is there hope for him if he continues with the chemotherapy? Am I wrongly condemning this form of "treatment"? In your eyes, is this something beneficial? Help me with the answer Lord. I know what I've seen, I know what I believe in my heart, but I need the wisdom that only you can provide on this.

"I have set my laws of nature upon the earth. The body is my temple. Think of it as a flowering and fruit-bearing plant which I have alluded to before. What do my plants need to thrive and give Me glory? They need air, water, sunshine, and good nutrient soil—all which I have provided. For man, the soil is threefold, the soil of the mind, the soil of the body, and the soil of the spirit. If there is a deficiency in one component, the plant will become 'diseased'. The solution, then, is to enrich the soils, and make sure there is enough water, air, and sunshine. Once the plant receives what it needs, I have provided mechanisms for it to overcome the 'disease' and to flourish.

Would you take a diseased plant and spray weed killer on it to get rid of the disease? With the very first spray, the plant cries out to me in groans and distress but is able to maintain life—even though the soils are still not enriched. With the 2nd spray, the plant cries out, but more weakly as its vitality and rigor are diminished. With each successive dose, there comes a point at which the plant cannot survive the onslaught. It is My law of nature. The plant is unable to bloom, withers, and dies an agonizing death. All of mankind are the flowers in My garden. *They themselves shall* *be like watered gardens, never again shall they languish.. (Jeremiah 31:12)*

Woe to the keepers of the garden, for they are no longer of Me. They no longer use the natural things I provide to 'enrich the soil'. *I was ready to respond to those who asked me not, to be found by those who sought me not. I said: Here I am, Here I am! (Isaiah 65:1)* **Go back to My ways and enrich the soils. My desire is for all of My plants to thrive and produce flowers—to exhibit My glory and splendor to the world. Amen."**

Thank you Lord. I never thought of these "treatments" in those terms, but you, in your wisdom, have helped me see clearly. Help us to "bloom" and to help others "bloom" for your glory. Pull us up out of the darkness for we are in quick-sand. Amen.

Enrich the Soil

God's words brought to mind the Magnolia tree in my front yard. We planted it 9 years ago when we purchased our home. It had never bloomed, much to my disappointment, and the leaves kept getting brown, burnt-looking areas on them. Some leaves would curl up and never looked right. Finally, I took sample leaves in to the local nursery and told the person there about the tree also having no blooms.

She said, "Ah, I know just what it needs. The soil is deficient in sulfur." She promptly retrieved a bag of sulfur and gave it to me with instructions. She said, "Use this sulfur as I have directed you to and I know that the tree will bloom. You wait and see." I was enriching the soil.

I spoke to the tree every day saying, "I need you to bloom as a sign to me—we can bloom together. All we need are the right nutrients. I know you can do it just like the other trees in the neighborhood! You are gorgeous!" Eight months later, that tree put out 5 beautiful blooms and I smiled and said, "Thank you—you are even more beautiful! I am going to bloom next!"

May 10
I dreamed that I could fly! No tethers, no one holding me back—pure flight and it felt so good—like floating. Thank you, Lord, for that wonderful experience! I saw a hawk flying and soaring with the thermals. What that must feel like!

"Diana, your time has come to soar like the hawk. You will fly higher and higher with a keen sense of my vision. Instead of hunting prey, as the hawk does, you will be looking for those that are lost and in need of help. You will be gathering souls for my kingdom. Each one of them is a frightened creature, in need of my help and salvation. They run, like scared rabbits, but do not know where to go or who to turn to. You shall show them the way, for you are on it. *...but those who hope in the Lord will renew their strength. They will soar on wings like eagles; they will run and not grow weary, they will walk and not grow faint. (Isaiah 30:41)*

Spread your wings—shake off all things unnecessary from your feathers and prepare to take flight. My path needs no roadway for I am the way." Lord, I will prepare, continue to pray, and look forward to "taking off" on your latest mission. Guide me, Jesus. Lead me. Continue to heal me. I remain humble in your sight.

"Soon, I will push you from the nest to go about the will of my Father. You have been fed and nurtured and now you are strong enough. The flower is opening its blossom. Amen."

Heavenly Pearls of Wisdom

Eat a mixture of cottage cheese and flaxseed oil. A little each day in the beginning would be good.

There's always a solution. Receive it and use it when God gives the answer.

God wants you to "bloom". When you do, you reveal His glory to the world.

After blooming, you will bear good fruit. Then the real work begins.

16
Changed Forever

May 11
May 6th was my 14th wedding anniversary with Lloyd. I am so grateful to be feeling healthy and good and to experience this. My thanks to you, Lord. May 7 was the 'National Day of Prayer'. We were asked to pray for the 7 seats of power, which are Government, Education, Military, Media, Business, Family, and Spiritual. EVERY day should be a day of prayer—not righteous prayer, in which we think we are better than any others, but humble prayer which seeks to put God's glory first. Lord, my prayer today is that all people in all areas above pray to have you reveal yourself to them—to glorify you and for themselves to recede. My prayer is also that people will humble themselves before you instead of circumstances having to humble them. I pray that our nation will always turn to you and never forget your mercy and goodness. May we never fear mixing Christianity with the 7 seats of power, for the world would see that we are your children and we would act humble in accordance with your Divine principles. **"My laws existed long before the laws of nations. I have placed those laws into the heart of every person. That is why they must continue to seek me within themselves. If individuals allowed me to work through them, businesses would be honest and**

not greedy, government would be just and not controlled by groups or those with money and influence, military might would only be needed for protection instead of being used as a political weapon by leaders, children would learn new meaning to their life in school, those responsible for communicating with the public would concentrate on stories of goodness and a sense of community instead of gore and opinion camouflaged as news, and families would work together with no violence all the while helping other families. *I will appoint peace your governor, and justice your ruler. No longer shall violence be heard in your land, or plunder and ruin within your boundaries. (Isaiah 60; 17-18)*

People fear having 'a religion' imposed upon them, yet fail to see that they are themselves imposing their internal chaos and lack of oneness with Me upon others instead. In preaching 'separation' from Me, they are fostering confusion, chaos, and darkness. It is in turning to me that peoples and nations are united. Pray for the illumination of the spirit for every individual. The original founders of your nation, who only had rudimentary candles, were much more 'illuminated' than your leaders of today, who have innumerable sources at their fingertips. Pray for Divine light to shine in all people. This reveals truth and truth shall guide and lead the way. Pray…Amen." *Let not your heart be troubled; you believe in God, believe also in me. (John 14:1)*

May 12

At the clinic, Melissa started me on some Nascent Iodine®, 3 drops 3 times a day. The brochure says that it helps with thyroid function, gets rid of metals, gets rid of chlorine, and many other benefits. I have been using it for several days and I love it! Many people who get diagnosed with cancer have low functioning thyroids and this will help provide the absorbable iodine that the body needs, especially since we don't eat enough fish from the sea to get the iodine we need.

> I will also see how this affects my body pH. I've been trying to keep it regulated because I know that is also very important.

Maintaining Body pH

What is pH? Very simply put, it is a measure of the number of acid or hydrogen ions present in a substance. It has a scale from 1, which is very acidic, to 14, which is very basic, and 7 is considered 'neutral pH', or an equal number of acidic and basic ions. An example of an acid is vinegar. An example of a base is soap or lye. Water is usually near a pH of 7. The pH of the blood in the body stays pretty close to 7.2 to 7.4 or slightly basic. The pH of the urine should stay slightly acidic, from 6.4-7.0. If the urine gets too acidic, irritation of the bladder usually occurs. If it becomes too basic, optimal conditions are set up for the growth of harmful bacteria. When I worked in the hospital, we always measured the pH of a patient's urine.

pH gives us a good indication of how the body is doing. I purchased some pH paper (also called litmus paper) from the grocery store in the health section and began to measure the pH of my urine and saliva daily. The one I have measures from 5.5 to 8.0. The saliva pH should also be in the range of approximately 6.4-6.6, or slightly acidic. In many diseased conditions, the pH of the body becomes too acidic, largely due to the types of foods being ingested. Robert Young, PhD, and Shelley Young state in their book, *THE PH MIRACLE, BALANCE YOUR DIET, RECLAIM YOUR HEALTH*, that "...overacidity interferes with life itself. It is at the root of all sickness and disease....Over acidity is also what's keeping you fat."[1] (In case you have that problem.) Sugar, processed foods, coffee, cheese, and beef make the body acidic, even though they are not acids themselves. Raw vegetables, olive oil, green tea, and most raw fruits make the body more alkaline. It is how the body processes the minerals in the foods that determines the resulting pH of the body. Too much fruit, which contains sugar, can also lead to more acid.

According to Pierce in *OUTSMART YOUR CANCER*[2], the diet should be three parts basic forming foods to one part acid forming foods. Yet, our typical diets are completely the opposite. Our goal is to enrich the soil of the body and when the pH gets out of balance, the opportunities for "diseased states" increase. According to the Youngs, the imbalance of blood pH leads to inflammation and irritation which sets the body up for invasion by bacteria, viruses, candida yeast, fungus, mold, and other disease. They also state that the overgrowth of yeast and fungi ferment sugar in the body to acetaldehyde which is converted in the liver to alcohol, making a person feel tired and mentally confused. This then leads to an exhaustive list of diseased conditions from PMS, to cancer, to asthma and depression, plus many more.[3] Go to an all-you-can-eat buffet and watch the amount of desserts people are taking.....maybe you are doing it too! Stop it! Whenever I see that my urine or saliva are becoming too acidic, I make sure that I get more basic forming foods. If the pH is getting too basic, higher than 7.4, I add back in some acid-forming foods. Pierce has a list of these foods in her book.

Patrick Quillin, in *BEATING CANCER WITH NUTRITION*[4], devotes several pages to the importance of pH. He states that cancer cells produce lactic acid from their uptake of sugar, thus making the body too acidic. This increased acidity helps more cancer cells to grow and a vicious cycle is set up. He says that you can tell if your body is too acidic by some outward signs. They are: 1) if your jewelry or your skin turns color when you wear it (for example, if it turns green), 2) you develop yeast or fungus infections, and 3) if mosquitoes stay away from you (I thought that would be a good thing, but I guess not!) He also states that healthy bacteria (probiotics) improve the pH of the colon.

Because lactic acid is the by-product of the cancer cells' anaerobic activity, not only does it lower the body pH, which makes the body very vulnerable to other infections, but the build-up of lactic acid leads to fatigue. That is why so many people who have a body riddled with cancer are so tired. (And I thought it was just lack of sleep.) The use of sugar for energy by cancer cells is a very inefficient system to get any energy to the rest of the body from regular food, thus leading to drastic weight loss in cancer patients. This is, in fact, a type of malnutrition.

It's probably a good idea to purchase some pH paper and regularly measure urinary and salivary pH. Then, based on the results, adjust the diet accordingly. This is such a simple step to take but so effective. One can also go on the internet and research what foods are acid-forming and which are base-forming. It's definitely worth the time.

May 17

We just returned from Iowa for my parent's 60th wedding anniversary, mom's 80th birthday, and dad's 86th birthday! Wow! Lord, please grant them many more blessings and thank you for them.

We had an open house for them and it was wonderful to see all of the relatives and meet new ones! The hardest part for me and yet endearing, was that at least 6 people wanted to talk with me about cancer. They either have cancer, had cancer, or know someone with cancer. Some were lost, and didn't know what to do. One has been told she's terminal and is taking chemotherapy because she doesn't know what other choices she has. My heart went out to each one of them. Now I know how Jesus felt when he came upon the masses and saw how they needed to be healed in either body, mind, spirit, or a combination of all three. He felt love and compassion.

As I looked into their eyes I saw sadness, fear, or despair. I wanted to heal each and every one of them instantly. Help me, Lord. I know you say not to take on certain burdens, but I pray for each person—that you will show them the way. Once again, I cry out to you. I will do as you direct me. Amen.

> On the plane, I sat next to a lady who works in a huge cancer clinic. What a coincidence! She was reading a book on therapeutic body massage and began to converse with me. When I found out where she worked I asked a few questions. What she told me about these treatment places was not pretty. God, where does it end?

A Mini-Interview

I don't recall the name of the woman that sat next to me on the plane but our conversation went something like this. She spoke to me first because I usually bury my head in a book on the plane and try to avoid conversation. I like to enjoy that time to read.

"Hello, are you heading to Texas or going on further?

"We're going to San Antonio, how about you?"

"I'm going back to California."

"I noticed you are reading a book on body massage."

"Yes, I'm not very happy with what I am doing now, so I thought I'd check this out."

"What line of work are you currently in?" She had my curiosity up now.

"I work in a cancer clinic." (I just about fell out of my seat. Why me, God? I did ask it this time.)

"That sounds interesting, at best," I said, somewhat cautiously. I didn't know where she was heading with this conversation.

"It's actually horrible and very depressing," she said sadly.

"In what way? You are trying to help people aren't you?"

"We say we are, but I know better. I know we are going to end up killing many of them and they look so lost and hopeless." Of course, at this point, I am sitting up pretty straight and paying close attention. Up to now in the conversation, she knew nothing of my experience. Without going into details, I told her about how I had started chemotherapy and then quit half-way through, and all else that had happened to me. Her reply was quite startling.

"It's a good thing you quit that stuff. You are so much better off. Because if someone didn't have a health problem besides cancer when they started chemotherapy, they will have some other problem by the time they're done! Especially diabetes! If they didn't have diabetes when they came in, we'll pretty much make sure they have it when their chemotherapy regimen is over. And they'll wonder where that came from." I was stunned, shocked, and so thankful that I never finished the prescribed traditional treatment.

"That's one of the reasons I can't take it anymore. I don't believe in what we are doing to people."

"That must be really hard on you."

"It's depressing and that is why I am going to find another line of work," she stated emphatically as she pointed to the open book in her lap.

"Do you have lots of patients?"

"We get 300 new patients a WEEK!" Did I hear her right? Did she just say 300?

"Whoa! That place must be huge!"

"We are one of the largest in California and I think they are going to open up another one."

"Well, I predict that you will find something more rewarding to do and this experience will only help you to embrace your new career with a new depth of joy and enthusiasm."

"Thanks, I sure hope so. I can't continue to look into the faces of the patients knowing what I know about the treatment."

"I wish you the best of luck, and it's been nice talking to you." And we got off the plane.

Even when we aren't actively seeking information, God brings us whatever information we need to hear, either something that contradicts what we have believed, something that confirms it, or something so new that it totally blows our mind. When we are seeking answers, they come from unexpected sources and at unexpected times. Someone once said that even when we are expecting something, it still comes when we least expect it and in the most unusual way. Thank you, Lord. That was definitely enlightening for me.

May 19
I was reflecting on the part of scripture in which a mother and two of the disciples of Jesus ask if they can sit on his right hand and his left hand in his "kingdom". Jesus asks his disciples in return, *Can you drink of the cup that I am going to drink? (Matthew 20:22)* They answered that they could. If my understanding is correct, the "cup" he was about to drink from was that of suffering and death. I wondered, could I drink of the cup? Would I be able to handle it? Did I even want to drink of it? And Jesus said to me in the midst of my musing, **"You have <u>already</u> drunk from it. Now, it is time for your resurrection. I do not ask for my people to drink from this cup, but when they do, and they remain faithful to me, resurrection comes. They must pray and sing praises, just as you have done. The old self dies, a new creation is born.**

Some have already sipped from the cup of sadness, anger, and suffering many times. However, they have turned from me rather than toward me. That cup, then, becomes the most bitter wine that has turned into vinegar, of which they repeatedly drink. Resurrection is only possible through ME. I will turn that vinegar into the sweetest wine.

I, the Lord Jesus, am the new covenant, the cup of the sweetest wine. Drink of me and you will be full of all that is good. You will thirst no more. I am always the answer. Amen."

Time to Sip Sweet Wine

No matter what we are going through, God desires to turn that situation into the "sweet wine." Let's claim that from his kingdom, to drink now of the sweet wine, and be free of the yoke of whatever had hold on us. I was more than ready for any fear to be over and to be restored to good health. I felt good. I now had to face the last hurdle—getting my blood tested. It had been a little over two years since the last CA-125. I knew that I was healed. God had told me DIRECTLY that I was healed, but for the rest of the world, I needed proof, which He understood.

When I went to the doctor to have the blood test ordered, he said, "Diana, do you have a plan in case these tests don't come out well?" "Yes, I do!" I replied, enthusiastically, all the while praying silently that I didn't need a back-up plan. "Well then, wait about a month since you just had your blood cell counts taken and we'll see how you do." I agreed and took the paperwork with the "orders" on them and put them in my car. A month went by and I kept looking at those papers on the seat of my car. Did I have the belief in God? Did I believe TOTALLY what he had said to me? What if I made it all up somehow? What kind of fool would people take me for then?

I vividly remember the reactions I received from various people when I announced that I was no longer going to chemotherapy and was embracing a holistic program. I've already spoken of what the oncologist had to say, but even a few of my friends told me they were disappointed that I had not chosen to finish the regimen. One of them is a retired physician. EVERY time she saw me she said, "Diana, you need to go finish that chemotherapy!" This came from someone who herself had colon cancer and received chemo. It left and then came back so she was undergoing a second chemo round. Another friend had said, "Diana, you need to do all that you can, including chemotherapy! I'm surprised that you don't want to do everything possible!"

Now, I understand how Noah must have felt when God told him there was a flood coming and to build an ark. People laughed at him and ridiculed him even though God had spoken to him directly and told him the flood was coming. In a way, I needed an "ark" to rise above all of the criticism I was being exposed to. I reminded myself of how the people quit laughing after several days of hard rain had fallen. There's a song that says, "Noah found grace in the eyes of the Lord and he left him high and dry." Lord, lift me up and let me be high and dry.

After I started the holistic program, many people looked at me doubtfully with raised eyebrows when I explained all that I was doing. One person said, "Well, even if you don't make it, at least you had a good life!" What kind of talk was that? I would have expected that kind of talk while taking chemotherapy, but not a natural approach! Others, especially health care professionals, would roll their eyeballs when I gave them the list of supplements I was taking. Then, I'd receive the "speech" about how they are unproven, dosages aren't guaranteed, that it was all quackery, they don't have research to back them up, etc. At least 2 or 3 people angrily told me that what I was doing was downright dangerous. ... *because of your long-suffering banish me not; know that for you I have borne insult. (Jeremiah 15:15)*

And, last, after I'd been on the program for about a year and a half, a couple of people would set me up and then "zing" me. They'd start off innocently asking, "How are you doing?" I'd reply, "I am doing absolutely great!" They'd look at me skeptically and say, "Well, you think you are doing great but do you have any proof?" That was the zinger. I had no "proof." My only proof was that I felt wonderful, had plenty of energy, and thought I looked ok, too.

May 20

Lord, it's time for my "proof." Please give me the courage to go and do what needs to be done. Give me the courage to believe in your words to me for all to see. I need the proof for your "book," the one you have told me to write. If I don't have the "proof," then all of this has been for naught and I will feel unable to win more souls for your kingdom. It's time for me to sip from the cup of your sweetest wine. I can taste it now. *I will raise the cup of salvation and call on the name of the Lord. (Psalm 116:13)* I feel so different than the person I was when this all first began, as if a totally new person has emerged—a better, brighter model of the first prototype. I feel like I am changed forever, never to return to my old ways of eating, thinking, believing, or praying. I might be missing a few body parts, but, I like this new me and it wouldn't have been possible without you, God. Thanks be to you. Amen.

May 21
It is done. I went to the laboratory with my papers in hand today and let them draw my blood. I took a few deep breaths to try and relax. The doctor has ordered a CA-125, which is to check for ovarian cancer, a CEA, which is a new test I've never heard of that tests for other cancers such as colon, lung, breast, etc, and the counts on all of my cells, the CBC.

I walked by the lab's blood drop off box and almost thought about waiting and retrieving my sample back out of there, but it was just a fleeting thought.

The blood is on its way to be tested. I can't stop it now. I must be brave and wait patiently for the results. I'm sort of glad that its Memorial Day holiday because I'm not in a hurry. At least the papers aren't sitting on my car seat any longer. OK, Lord....take the car and here we go.

Heavenly Pearls of Wisdom

Measure your body pH. Try to keep it between 6.4 and 7.2
Conduct your own interviews. It's amazing the truth you will uncover unwittingly.
Sip the sweet wine. Taste and see the goodness of the Lord.

17
Light Unto the Darkness

May 22
I talked with my sister recently and asked how Myron was doing. He is doing very well considering that almost 2 years ago, the doctors said they could do no more for him and basically told him to enjoy what little time he had left. Myron still has the stomach tube for feeding since his esophagus hasn't opened up yet. Joann has him on a substance called Protocel™ and I think it may have saved his life. Lord, thank you for the resources you provide. I pray that Myron is healed and will continue to manifest your glory. He has certainly been an inspiration to me. He doesn't know it, but he is. Thanks, Myron.

Alternative Treatments

There are so many alternative treatments that it would be impossible to cover them here. Each person is led to the information as they need it. The best resource for me was the book I mentioned earlier, *Outsmart Your Cancer*. Tanya Pierce researched several alternative methods and interviewed many people for her book. She was astounded at what she found because so many people had been cured permanently of all forms of cancer.

A few of the treatments she covers are as follows: The Hoxsey Therapy, Essiac Tea, The Gerson Method (which the clinic I attend is partly based on), Laetrile (a concentrated form of B_{17}), Dr. Kelley's Enzyme Therapy, Protocel™, Oxygen Therapy (ozone, hyperbaric oxygen, or hydrogen peroxide), flaxseed oil and cottage cheese, 714X, and Cesium High pH Therapy. My sister Joann, after reading all of these, chose Protocel™.

Protocel is a liquid formula that is taken by mixing a very small amount (1/8 to 1/4th teaspoon) into water and taking it four or five times a day. There are two kinds, Protocel 23 and Protocel 50, depending on the type of cancer. It does not need refrigeration, can go through the airport scanners, and has a long shelf life. It is also VERY affordable—about $55-75 per month—tons cheaper than chemotherapy and with no toxic properties. It works basically by lowering the voltage of the body's cells to the point where cancer cells literally fall apart and healthy cells stay intact. Pierce states that when the cancer cells break down in people using Protocel, they may see mucous-like material in their urine or feces as the body rids itself of the "waste." She devotes four chapters of her book to this therapy and explains it well.[1] My sister orders the Protocel from the internet because she and Myron live in a very small town on a farm.

I met another lady recently whose husband is doing well undergoing Ozone treatment. She also stated that he had been given a terminal diagnosis but was extremely pleased at his progress. Cancer cells do not thrive well in an oxygen-rich environment. Therefore, when oxygen is forced into the tissues, such as with hyperbaric oxygen treatments, the cancer cells may be completely destroyed.

Some alternative treatments are very expensive and therefore, are not available to many people, since, at this time, insurance does not cover them. Someday, hopefully, that will change as people see more and more results with their friends and relatives getting healed.

Unfortunately, these methods are not sought out until conventional medicine has given up on them and made them even more ill. That fact makes gathering enough positive data very difficult. Even with positive data, as you will see when researching many of these methods, the data is squelched because drug companies or some other entity either cannot make money off of them or feel threatened by the results.

May 25
It is Memorial Day (sort of, but not really, since they changed it to a Monday). I remember those who have sacrificed for me and my country, including Matthew Kuglics. I talked with his mom, Donna. It's been two years since Matthew was killed in Iraq and the pain is just as sharp as it was then. Every time June 5 comes around, she, Les, and Emily will stop whatever they are doing and remember their brave, fallen hero. My heart still goes out to them as they try to go on living their lives and taking care of his dog, Hunter. My prayers are with all who have fallen, as well as their families and descendants. We are so fortunate to be here. Thank you, Lord.

May 26
I was gone a good portion of the day and when I returned, I listened to the message on our answering machine instruct me to call my doctor's office concerning my laboratory test results. The day of reckoning had indeed arrived. Was it to be the resurrection I had been promised? I knew it had to be good news—it just had to be. I will always remember the conversation when I called them back.

"Medical group, how can I help you?" I wanted to say, you can tell me that I'm healed.

"This is Diana Fidone-Griggs and I'm calling about my lab results."

"Just a moment—please hold." If the doctor's voice came on the line, it might not be the best news; if the assistant came on the line, it was no big deal. I'd learned this from other experiences. The seconds ticked by as I waited patiently.

"This is Heather, how can I help you?" I repeated my request. "Hmmm…let's see….can you hold?" Good grief…I wanted to be finished with waiting on a medical figure (that we have been indoctrinated with) to tell if all was well. This test is not for me to know whether or not I am healed, but for all who know me and are doubtful, along with the doctors. When Jesus was at the temple, a leper approached him and asked to be healed. *After Jesus healed him, he said to the leper, "See that you don't tell this to anyone. But go, show yourself to the priest and offer the sacrifices that Moses commanded for your cleansing, as proof for them." (Mark 1:44)* This will be proof for the "priest."

"Yes, I'll hold." More 'hold' music played while I waited.

"Here are your results." It was the same voice which was a positive sign. "The CA-125 is 21 and up to 21 is normal, your CEA is 0.4 and normal is less than 2.5. Your white count is still low at 2.7 and normal is 4-10."

Although I was not tied to this number and knew that I was healed, I wanted to dive into the phone and give her a big hug! "That is expectedly good news! Thank you so much!"

"You're welcome and have a nice day." Have a nice day? I'm having a nice LIFE! Thank you, God! *You have given me health and life; thus is my bitterness transformed into peace. You have preserved my life from the pit of destruction. (Isaiah 38:16-17)*

God has won the victory for me! *We went through fire and flood, but you brought us to a place of great abundance. (Psalm 66:12)* These are the results the Lord promised!

At dinner, Lloyd and I toasted the results with a clink of wine glasses, thanking the Lord, praying, and giving him praise. I broke down and sobbed and it felt good to cry tears of joy for the first time in a long time. Thank you, Lord, for my resurrection from the darkness. Thank you for the proof of your glory! You promised this and I had often been weak, but you saw me through. You are a most merciful and compassionate God! *The living, the living give you thanks, as I do today. (Isaiah 38:19)* Amen.

"What I have given to you I offer to all—I offer My love. It will appear to them in many forms. It has appeared to you as healing. You were healed long ago, but did not yet fully believe. If others will only believe in Me, what they need <u>will</u> appear." *With age-old love I have loved you; so I have kept my mercy toward you. (Jeremiah 31:3)*

I love you, my God. I humbly give myself to you—I praise your name. I give you unending thanks. I bow before your greatness.

"That is all that I ask—heavenly hosts rejoice in your joy of me. Now, prepare yourself. Finish my book and set about my business."

Lord, I will gladly do as you have asked. *How can I repay the Lord for all good done for me? (Psalm 116:12)* Amen.

Energy Sources

Lately, I have been using a product called Nascent® Iodine. It costs less than $40 per bottle and I only take 3 drops, 3 times a day in a little water. The benefits of Nascent® Iodine listed in the company information are these: 1) increases cellular metabolism, 2) nourishes the thyroid gland, 3) naturally elevates the body's pH levels, 4) aids in the excretion of toxic fluoride, bromine, and chlorine, 5) assists chelation of heavy metals mercury, cadmium, and lead, 6) supports healthy breast tissue, prostate, and ovaries, 7) increases antioxidant activity and immune system function, and 8) assists in regulating mood. It has been remarkable for me, added to all of the other things I have been doing. My energy levels are higher than ever and my body temperature is staying consistently warm. I used to get very cold, especially in the air conditioning of some restaurants and offices, but now I stay nice and warm, with no jacket! What a change this has been for me. My levels of things the holistic clinic measures have been good also! I'm glad I gave it a try! Of course, if someone is allergic to iodine, this product does not seem like a viable possibility.

Another product that the clinic had me take when I first arrived there after chemotherapy is called "Liquid Needle®" Brown ReBalancer. It is a form of water containing light-energized molecules that carry light wave frequencies to areas of the body. This seems to provide energy and strength to areas of the body that are most in need. A few drops are added to water and it is tasteless and odorless.

None of these items may bring about healing by themselves, but together with other foods and supplements, I believe they have worked synergistically to bring my body back into balance.

June 1
I am still so grateful for my test results. **"Diana, it is not over, for My work has just begun in you. Now, the flower blooms and manifests My glory. Then, comes the fruit—the fruit that will feed others. Come, we have work to do. Take My hand.** *I, the Lord, have called you for the victory of justice, I have grasped you by the hand; I formed you, and set you as a covenant of the people, a light for the nations. (Isaiah 42:6)* **The path is still there—the one I set out for you long ago—my path. Walk it—I will set the pace and I shall lay out the tasks."** *Blessed be God, who did not refuse me the kindness I sought in prayer. (Psalm 66:20)*

Only "Give In" to Truth

When listening to a radio station one day, I heard the host ask a famous person (can't remember who) what the main ingredient of any success is. This applies to any situation such as health, money, relationships, careers, etc. Or, to put it another way, he was also asked what one ingredient makes people fail. As I was listening, I tried to come up with the answer and nothing came to mind, except maybe belief that success is possible. I will always remember this answer because it was so simple, yet so profound.

The person stated that the cause of peoples' failures is that they give in to their own excuses. Bingo! Once I heard this astounding revelation, I began to listen intently to what my friends, clients, relatives, acquaintances, or people I met by chance, were saying. I was at lunch with some friends and one of them said, "I can't do that because of my condition." The "giving in" takes many forms but the basic message is one of "I can't do this because... or I don't want to do that because..." This is a perfect example of two gigantic mistakes that people make. The first mistake is to decide to take ownership of a disease or condition and make it their own. The second mistake is to give in to the excuse(s) they are making of what is holding them back.

I heard the same types of excuses when people would ask me what I was doing in the holistic program I was following. I would excitedly tell them all the things I was doing and they would respond with, "I couldn't do all of the things necessary to follow such a program. It's too much work." Or they would give some other reason, but the result is still the same. What are they doing? They are not only making an excuse, but they are <u>internalizing</u> that excuse and making it a part of their inner self. Once it is internalized, the subconscious mind will make sure that it remains in place. People would do well to examine what they are saying and instead of giving in to their excuses, to give in to the truth that all things are possible with the Lord—<u>all</u> things.

I saw a bird with only one leg the other day and it reminded me of the "don't give-in–to-excuses" message. The bird did not say, "I'm handicapped, so I can't look for food or compete with the other birds, so I guess I'll just lie down and give up." He was amidst the other birds, pecking away and fighting for his food with the rest of them. He gave in to the truth that he deserved to be there and was able to live and thrive just like the rest of them. That's why children are an inspiration. If no one tells them they can't do something (like parents or teachers sometimes do), they are in the midst of other children, giving it all they've got.

There are countless stories of people in the Bible attempting to give in to their excuses, but God always dismissed those or would over-ride them. God did not fall for it when his people made excuses. The call of Moses is a clear indication of this. God told Moses, *I have witnessed the afflictions of my people in Egypt, and heard their cry of complaint against their slave drivers, so I know well what they are suffering. (Exodus 3:7).* Then He said, *Come now! I will send you to the Pharaoh to lead my people, the Israelites, out of Egypt. But Moses said to God, Who am I that I should go to Pharaoh and lead the Israelites out of Egypt?* (1st excuse) *God answered, I will be with you...* Then Moses tried a 2nd excuse, *But...when I go to the Israelites....and say... the God of your fathers has sent me...if they ask me, what is his name? what do I tell them? God replied, I am who am...I AM sent me to you. (Exodus 3: 11-19)* So, Moses tried a 3rd excuse, *But... suppose they will not believe me, nor listen to my plea? (Exodus 4:1)* God didn't fall for this and instructed Moses to do some things to demonstrate the power of God. Even then, Moses tried a 4th excuse, *If you please, Lord, I have never been eloquent, neither in the past, nor recently, nor now that you have spoken to your servant... (Exodus 4:10)* Do you see the subtle "I can't because..." excuses on the part of Moses for why he can't confront Pharaoh? And God said, *Go, then! It is I who will assist you in speaking... (Exodus 4:12)* And Moses tried for a 5th time to get out of it, *If you please, Lord, send someone else! (Exodus 4: 13)* But God would have none of it— no giving in to excuses, just go! He even got a little angry with Moses and finally Moses gave in to the truth of what needed to occur and the plan was carried out. Whew!

It would have been easy for me to accept what the doctor said and just give in. It might be easier for some to take chemo so they don't have to change anything else. But I refused to accept someone else's limitations on my life or on the power of the Lord. I refused to give in to the excuse of some disease that someone else said I had. I gave in to the truth that I could and would manifest wholeness once again.

The Path to Truth

Each person is on a path to discover the truth—whatever truth is needed for their unfolding as a flower, so they can bear good fruit. There are 7 steps to discovering and living each truth. The steps are outlined in the following paragraphs.

Step 1 is skepticism. When people hear or see something new or something that contradicts their experience or beliefs, they are extremely skeptical. This is a normal reaction and is part of our protective mechanism, to keep close to us that which we currently hold true based on our knowledge and experience. If it is truth one is learning, then at the present moment, that person is in "darkness" related to that truth. Sometimes, people prefer the darkness.

Let's use the life of Jesus as an example. When he began speaking in the temple with such knowledge and authority at a young age, people, especially the elders, spoke out with skepticism. "*Where did this man get this wisdom and miraculous powers?", they asked. "Isn't this the carpenter's son?" (Matthew 13:54-55)* They were uncomfortable with the fact that he was shedding "new light" on the scriptures, their beliefs, and their practices. *Then the disciples came to him and asked, "Do you know the Pharisees were offended when they heard this?" (Matthew 15:12)*

Step 2 is denial. People may hear the truth again and again or see it demonstrated, but they out and out deny it exists. The "light" is starting to hurt their eyes, like those of a mole coming out of a cave. In the case of Jesus, they stated, "*It is by the prince of demons that he drives out demons." (Matthew 9:34)* They decided that they would brand him "evil" as a form of denial. Furthermore, he was claiming to be the Son of God, and there was no way this could be true—no, not the carpenter's son.

Step 3 is sabotage. If people are conflicted or feel threatened when exposed to the truth, they don't want to change their beliefs and thinking or their resultant behaviors. They have settled comfortably into their "velvet rut," as one of my former bosses used to say. Now, people are definitely bothered and are now thinking, "Turn that darn light off! It's too bright and getting brighter!" It's time to act. The first act of sabotage against Jesus was to try and attack him in the temple. He had to run and escape the crowd. But the worst act of sabotage was yet to come; *But the Pharisees went out and plotted how they might kill Jesus. (Matthew 12:14) Wanting to satisfy the crowd (interested in sabotage) Pilate released Barabbas to them. He had Jesus flogged and handed him over to be crucified. (Mark 15:15)*

Step 4 is seeking proof. If something is true, people demand proof before they will accept this new notion. Where is that light coming from? How can we trust its source? The proof came when Jesus rose from the dead. But, even then, the church elders paid off the Roman soldiers to say that his followers came and stole the body. However, that excuse didn't work for long. His followers were also mystified, but the angel at the tomb told them the "real story." *The angel said to the women, "Do not be afraid, for I know that you are looking for Jesus, who was crucified. He is not here; he has risen, just as he said." (Matthew 28:5-6)* And the word spread like wildfire.

The apostles were still frightened and had locked themselves into a room. And who should appear as "proof" but the Master himself, Jesus. He scared the wits out of them at first. But, then what happened next? *Jesus came and stood among them and said, "Peace be with you!" Then he showed them his hands and side (John 20:19-20),* as if to say, "See, here's your proof. It's really me." One disciple wasn't in the room, Thomas, and he refused to believe after all of the rest of the apostles said they had seen Jesus. He demanded proof for himself. He boldly stated, *"Unless I see the nail marks in his hands, and put my finger where the nails were, and put my hand into his side, I will not believe it." (John 20:25)* A week later, when Thomas was with the group and they were once again behind locked doors, Jesus appeared to them again. *Then he said to Thomas, "Put your finger here; see my hands. Reach out your hand and put it into my side. Stop doubting and believe." (John 20:27)* Unfortunately, Thomas represents the masses of people who refuse to believe anything without proof. They are truly "doubting Thomases."

Therefore, when one is faced with an illness, it is extremely difficult for some to believe that they can and will be healed. They want proof that something works. The drug companies and medical personnel play on this by stating that there is no proof that holistic or alternative methods, supplements, or herbs actually work. Yet, when proof is gladly provided, they deny it and then sabotage the carrier of the news. They discredit the results and kill the credibility of the messenger.

Wanting proof is also why people can't believe it when someone is healed and says that God was instrumental in the healing. There is no proof of that except what Jesus did while on earth. Even when a "flow of grace," which we call a miracle, occurs, the scientific community will try to find a logical explanation for the immediate improvement. Miracles and natural healing don't fit into the medical and logical framework.

Step 5 is <u>acceptance</u>. This takes longer, but if the belief or principle is truly the truth, it brings with it a new peace. The light doesn't seem to be going away. In fact, people now rather like its beautiful flame. Once the apostles became accustomed to the idea that Jesus had risen from the dead and was now hanging out with them again for at least 40 days, they accepted all that he had told them about himself. When he showed his wounds to Thomas, Thomas accepted the entire package and summed it up succinctly when he said, *My Lord and My God! (John 20:28)* The apostles had accepted that he was God manifested as a man or the Son of God.

Step 6 is enlightenment. Not only is the truth accepted but the "aha" moment occurs in which it is internalized and the person gains a deeper and more profound sense of it. Jesus spent those last 40 days working with the disciples and allowing them to become certain and unwavering in their new understanding of all that he had revealed to them.

An example of enlightenment occurs after Jesus ascends into heaven. Peter was left in charge of the new group of believers. One day he and John were going into the temple when a cripple approached them for money. Peter took him by the hand and instantly, his legs and ankles straightened up and he began to dance around. The people were astonished and came running over to see what had happened. Peter asked, "Why does this surprise you?" He showed his level of enlightenment when he said to the crowd, *By faith in the name of Jesus, this man whom you see and know was made strong. It is Jesus' name and the faith that comes through him that has given this complete healing to him, as you can all see. (Acts 3:16)* He was trying to say, "Look, I get it—why can't you all get it?"

Step 7 is the final stage of zeal. People understand and are set afire with a passion ignited in them to share the truth with others who are still "in the dark." They are thinking, "Let me bring the light to the caves of the others! Wait until they experience this!" People who have acquired this level of enthusiasm for any ideal are called zealots. Their mission is to bring the truth to the skeptics.

On the day of Pentecost, the apostles received the Holy Spirit as tongues of fire. From that moment on, they were on fire and ready to preach the word in many languages to the "skeptics" of their day. They confidently began to talk to the crowd that had gathered since they were all speaking in different languages. People in the crowd even accused them of being drunk! Peter rose and gave a lengthy speech which the people listened to intently. *Therefore, let all Israel be assured of this: God has made this Jesus, whom you crucified, both Lord and Christ. (Acts 2:36)* Then, they asked, "What are we to do with this information?" And Peter said, *Repent and be baptized, every one of you, in the name of Jesus Christ for the forgiveness of your sins. And you will receive the gift of the Holy Spirit. (Acts 2:38)*

The progression from criticism to zeal will hopefully unfold slowly and carefully in the skeptics, like a flower, just as it has in me. I guess I could now be called a zealot for the truth as I have discovered it through research and in communion with our Lord. It is not a secret. It is not only for me. The truth is for all and God reveals Himself when people invite him in and then wait patiently. Where are you in this process?

May the Lord bless you and work in you to bear wonderful fruit. May you be ignited by the fire of God's mercy and love, and allow the truth to be burned into your very core. The flame will roar and crackle as you become the flame itself. Once the flame is burning brightly in you, may you send out, into the darkness, many "sparks."

June 2

I had a dream last night. I was in what appeared to be a futuristic station, like a light monorail, but much more sophisticated. Everything was white—white walls, white floors, white transportation vehicle.

I boarded the vehicle and realized two things. I didn't know where I was going and I had no luggage! I'd left my luggage at the hotel! I panicked. But, then I calmed down and thought that the hotel might collect it up and send it to me or that I could just buy new clothes! (Any excuse to go shopping!)

I prayed about the meaning of this strange dream and heard this answer, **"Diana, where you are going, you need**

take nothing for I shall provide all. You do not need any luggage from the past for it serves no purpose and it is only now that matters. Do not worry about where you are going for I am in charge. Sit back, relax, and marvel at what is to come."

But, Lord, what if I don't know the way?

"I am the way."

Once again, I put my trust in you. Thank you, Lord. May I bear fruit wherever you lead me and may I give glory to your name forever on bended knee. Amen.

Heavenly Pearls of Wisdom

Research alternative methods. If one is right for you, you will be led to it.

Get energy back into your body. It is necessary for life's functions.

Only give in to truth. Don't make excuses for anything that is not of God to be part of you.

Discover your stage of truth. When you do, you can remove any blockages to receiving God's grace of enlightenment and zeal and be healed.

18
Arriving At a New Place

June 14
I sent an e-mail out to my friends to let them know that I now had test results that showed healing and have already received two phone calls from friends that they referred to me. O, Lord, I want to help so many people, and yet all I can do is give them the very beginning. They have to connect with you to find what will be best for them. **"You are helping them, Diana. You are bringing them to Me and to the truth. They have the desire to be led to it and their hearts are ready. I have heard and answered their call.**

Whenever I bring people together, they have each answered the other's prayer. If people only realized how closely they are connected in my Divine spirit, there would be no indifference toward others. Part of your mission is to show others their connectedness to me first, then to each other. This is spoken of by Paul as the body of Christ. We are all one body. Amen." *Just as each of us has one body with many members, and these members do not all have the same function, so in Christ we who are many form one body, and each member belongs to all the others. (Romans 12:4-5)*

June 15
I drew great inspiration from Mark, Chapter 14. It's time for the apostles to have the Passover meal, in which they celebrate the

angel of death passing them over while they were in Egypt, and the first born of each Egyptian was killed to convince Pharaoh to release the Israelites who had been their slaves.

For the Passover meal, Jesus instructed them to go into the city, find a man who was carrying a jar of water, follow him, and ask him where the great room was for the Teacher and them to eat. *He will show you a large upper room, furnished and prepared. Make preparations for us there. The disciples left, went into the city, and found things just as Jesus had told them. (Mark 14:14-16)*

I've heard that passage at least 50 times in my life and the significance of it was inspirational. The room was already prepared! Even though the apostles didn't know it, the room was ready! Why had the man with the water jar gotten the room ready? What moved him to do it? Did he think to himself, "I'll get the room ready in case I have guests tonight?"

God, you are truly awesome! If I believe that you have already prepared something wonderful for me, it appears at its appointed time! Whatever I need, it's already there!

"All that I prepare for my people is done with love. I love them so dearly, but I myself must abide by the laws I have set in place. They who await and expect my goodness and mercy with eager anticipation shall indeed see it made manifest in the proper order. Many times, the receiving of it depends on the state of their heart—are they giving me thanks and praise? If so, then their hearts are open and ready. If not, then their hearts are hardened and not ready.

If they come to me, I will make them ready and then they will receive grace. Once grace abounds, all good comes to them and from them. It is always prepared and ready. When they receive, the circumstances that result will be to their delight. When they delight in Me, they receive even more. I have prepared all. Amen."

June 17

The more I read my Bible, the more amazed I become at all of the truths and concepts of the Spirit contained in the words of scripture. I was praying, telling God that each one of the stories of Him is so fascinating, and how different insights arrive with each story through Him. For example, Jesus asked the disciples, "Who do people say I am?" The other apostles were taking guesses, but only Peter got it right when he said, *You are the Christ, the Son of the living God. Jesus replied, Blessed are you Simon son of Jonah, for this was not revealed to you by man, but by my Father in Heaven. (Matthew 16:16-17)* Lord, thank you so much for all of the times you reveal yourself to me and us! Please continue to guide me and teach me your ways and truths. I am so eager to learn of you and to please you. Amen.

"The scriptures contain many stories and each story has many other stories and lessons within it, waiting to be discovered by those who love Me. I put those lessons into the hands of the holy ones who wrote the words. All of the writers speak of my Kingdom, which man has trouble grasping. The rules of My Kingdom are not the same as those of earth. Earth is but a shadow of what is to come to those who have faith in My goodness and love. My Son prepared the way and those who believe shall follow it. When all veils are lifted and complete understanding dawns, they are ready to enter. Continue to prepare so that you, too, will be ready when the appointed time comes."

June 21

I heard the birds singing so beautifully in our trees this morning. I told the Lord thank you for the wonderful sounds of nature that he created just for us. I don't dare open our windows at night because we live near a quarry and in the middle of the night, the heavy trucks start the grinding journey to wherever they are going. The noise they make grates on the nerves. But, the sounds of the birds and nature during the day are so pleasing to the ear. I wonder why that is? **"It is how I call each person to me."** *He calls his own sheep by name and leads them out. When he has brought out all* *his own, he goes out ahead of them, and his sheep follow him because they know his voice. (John 10:3-4)*

"I sing sweetly to each one, whisper in their ear, and call them by name. Those who hear come to my table and then we fly. Those who turn a deaf ear wander aimlessly, unable to take flight. Because they focus on the world, they may hop up a few times as a bird does, but they always come back down and never fly.

Hear the sweet call. I am calling you to do wondrous things in my name. You have the power. Do not be afraid. Do not doubt. You have it. It is with the power of my wings under yours that you fly. Then, the Holy Spirit sustains you and you continue your flight. It is time to fly. I will direct you. No one shall grab your leg or keep you down again. I shall see to it. Straight as the crow flies is your path."

God Sings You to Him

God whispers and sings to us! A most wondrous beauty! I never thought of God using the sounds of nature to "call" us. *Then I heard every creature in Heaven and on earth and under the earth and on the sea, and all that is in them, singing: To him who sits on the throne and to the lamb be praise and honor and glory and power, forever and ever! (Revelation 5:13)* A few days later, Lloyd and I rented the movie *Australia* with Nicole Kidman and Hugh Jackman.[1] In the story is a half-breed Aborigine child living on a ranch. When Nicole's character, Mrs. Boss as they call her, arrives on the ranch, he looks her squarely in the eyes and very tenderly, but with confidence and conviction, announces, "I sang you to me." He knew without a doubt that after meeting her, his life was going to change drastically. He knew, from the wisdom taught to him by his elders, the elements of the spirit world. He knew that if he "sang her" to him, that song reached across time, land, and sea. He and Mrs. Boss are pulled apart by circumstances, but once again he tells her with conviction, "I will sing you back to me," which he eventually does.

God is singing you to Him.....listen!! Do you hear? Then, we, in turn, sing his praises and sing Him to us. *I will sing to the Lord all my life, I will sing praise to my God as long as I live. (Psalm 104:33)* Sing him to you. Sometimes, I might be in the middle of cleaning the bathroom (a job I truly hate), and I suddenly break out in song to God. I often wonder why I do that. Am I singing Him to me or am I already feeling His presence because He sang me to Him? Either way, life is abounding.

June 22

I did a real estate market analysis for someone and because I did not include one parameter, it caused a small problem for the person for whom I performed it. I agonized over this for days because I feared that I would lose credibility in this person's eyes who I value very much as a friend, and I felt humiliated. My skin has broken out in a rash with fluid-filled little bumps all over. Lord, I recognize that this is a manifestation of the agitation of my inner being. I ask you to turn my cup of vinegar into sweet wine. I ask for your help, Lord. I know that you are the one and only source we turn to. **"I gladly take your burden, Diana. But, give it ALL to me. Offer me not only the situation itself, but your feelings and emotions, for they are at the core of your suffering. Ask me to replace those feelings with love and grace. Pride, humiliation, anger, and agitation have no place in My Kingdom. Imagine an empty box that I bring to you. Fill it with those feelings and watch as I close the lid, remove the box from you, and toss it into the flames. The fire of my love consumes them and they lose their power over you and become the fire of my love. Your only goal is to please me. When you hope to please others, situations will cause great agony. You were simply trying to help another and that is very pleasing to me. I shall take care of the rest and turn this into goodness, because you have turned to me.**

Now, go forth happily, like a child who soon forgets that he has fallen down and scraped his knee as soon as he receives consolation from his mother. He resumes his play as if nothing had happened. It is forgotten. Amen."

Thank you Lord. May this "eruption" of negative feelings be swallowed up in the cool soothing love that you provide. Then, I know that the eruptions of my skin shall disappear. Blessed be my Lord. Forgive my pride. If I had no pride to begin with, I wouldn't have to agonize over losing it. Amen.

June 23
Sure enough, just as the Lord promised, the situation worked out well. Whew and thank you Lord! The rash and bumps are still prominent, but I know they will go away soon.

June 26
Farah Fawcett, a well-known actress, passed away yesterday from cancer. It is so sad—another needless death. O Lord, for the 100th time, my very being cries out to you for an end to this darkness, disease, and destruction. She was only 62 years old. Why does this still go on? When will it end?

"The answer is already among you. I have provided it, but evil men have squelched the information. The truth is available to all, but they do not seek it. When enough people seek the truth, all will change. To all things there is truth and there are lies. Many accept the lies because a lie always appears as the easier way. Therein is its deception. A lie is accepted by those who do not truly know me, the Christ.

'Seek and ye shall find' means to seek the truth. I am truth. *When you look for me, you will find me. Yes, when you seek me with all your heart, you will find me with you... (Jeremiah 29:13-14)* **Truth will be revealed to those who ask me to reveal it to them, whether it is the truth about a situation, a person, or a treatment. But, if one never seeks, one dies in darkness. Continue to seek, Diana. You are becoming**

enlightened but you shall never stop seeking. Those who continue to seek obtain the Kingdom. Amen." *So, I say to you, ask and it will be given to you, seek and you will find; knock and it will be opened to you. (Luke 11:9)*

July 1
Lord, I have been thinking about how grateful I am that you have healed me, but also wondering how I can be strengthened and go forth in the world with confidence that this will never happen again. **"With the help of My grace, you will learn to recognize the absence of goodness (which is evil) and love (which is fear) in all seductive and deceptive forms. Offer your prayers to Me to learn of your spiritual weaknesses and for them to be banished by Me. This is the beginning of spiritual strength."**

Recognizing Unholy Suggestions

Knowing that I was healed was wonderful, but for anyone who has experienced the darkness of serious ill health, healing is only the beginning of the process. We long for assurance that the healing is permanent—not short-lived. We desire to know and believe that whatever it was that appeared is gone and never ever will return. I realized that I was not yet at that level of confidence.

Doesn't that seem odd? That I could be given faith, through the grace of God, to be healed and not have enough faith left over to remain healed? I have to ignore the history of cancer among the people. More and more I heard, "So and so had cancer, went through chemo, was pronounced in remission, and 6 months later, it's come back. Now it's in this organ and that organ...." How can I be surrounded by this kind of talk and thinking and not soak it in, like my friend Maggie did? The boiling oil is still around me.

God was telling me to be alert, to know that I'm still surrounded by the boiling oil of doubt and fear that something could come after me a second time. I needed to become impervious and impenetrable to the fear. O, Lord, take my weaknesses and replace them with strengths and confidence. You are the answer to all. Remove any fear every time I get an ache or pain. Remove fear when I hear others tell of the relapses of friends or relatives. Replace that fear with confidence in your love—to trust that not only is all well, but that all will remain well. Comfort me as the mother does and send me back out to play in the world. May I never again think about any kind of physical, mental, or spiritual wound as even being possible!

Lloyd and I viewed the movie *Madagascar 2: Escape to Africa*.[2] I had to laugh at the antics of Melman (I'll call him Mel.), the giraffe in the story. He and his pals end up in Africa after escaping from the New York City Zoo. One day, Mel and the other giraffes are all standing together when one of the giraffes tells the others that Mel has some spots on his neck. Oh, no! The other giraffes quickly concur that Mel certainly does have dreaded spots. He becomes very concerned and then alarmed when one after another, his buddies tell him that he is doomed. *Even from your own number men will arise and distort the truth... (Acts 20:30)* They stated that the previous witch doctor giraffe with the same spots had gone off to die.

They figured that Mel probably had about 4 days to live. In the next scene, Mel is lying down in a deep hole in the ground (that he dug for himself?) with only his head sticking out, convincing himself that he feels bad, waiting to die. To anyone who passes by, he restates his condition and reaffirms his damning situation and illness. *...because every man's own word becomes his oracle and so you distort the words of the living God, the Lord almighty, our God. (Jeremiah 23:36)* It was so hard for me to not be like Mel at times.

A doctor tells us that we have some serious condition or cancer. He or she follows that up by saying that we only have a limited time to live no matter what they do, and we blindly and automatically accept and embrace this as the absolute truth. We immediately go and dig our own hole and step in by accepting whatever they tell us to do. We are so full of fear that we forget to ask God what to do. I know because I was in the hole for a while. We have unknowingly given in to the diagnosis and its prognosis and said to God, "Well, I guess it's over, you're powerless, and I'm on my way to my heavenly home".

Julien, the king of the lemurs, passes by Mel in the hole and Mel states that he regrets he hasn't loved and enjoyed life to the fullest. Julien tells him that he ought to get out and enjoy what he's always wanted to do. Mel immediately agrees and, with a renewed sense of purpose and great energy, rises up out of the hole, and runs off to find the love of his life. Mel later finds out that the dreaded spots are harmless and simply normal giraffe spots.

This is a powerful message that illustrates that things are not always what people assume them to be. It is our interpretation and acceptance of a situation that makes that situation real for us. The other giraffes had assumed that Mel was going to bite the dust because they thought that's what had happened to another giraffe. Mel had accepted what his friends told him and yet, it was only an imagined situation with no real basis.

...God is light, and in him there is no darkness at all. If we say, 'We have fellowship with him,' while we continue to walk in darkness, we lie and do not act in truth. (1 John 1:5-6) When he was made aware of the truth, he was able to give up the 'lie' about his condition. If only he had recognized the suggestions of the other giraffes as just unholy suggestions, he would have been so much better off. But, not recognizing this, he reacted, became fearful and discouraged, expecting death instead of life.

My prayer is that you and I will not 'react' to anything that tries to suggest anything less than perfect health and well being to us. With the help of the Lord, I will recognize when something or someone is trying to invade my consciousness. Then, knowing that God is all in all, I shall ask him to remove these suggestions and fears and replace them with trust and confidence. If He is for me, who can be against?

July 2
The sparrows have built a nest in the tree by our second story window! What a wonder of nature that is! Thank you, Lord, for giving me the privilege to see this. The sparrow (I don't know if it's male or female) is guarding that nest with his or her very life. Any bird that comes near is immediately and vehemently chased off with much fluttering and angry bird sounds. **"This represents my directive to you and to others. Ask me to guard your innermost being from all attempts by anyone or anything to come at you, just as the sparrow guards its nest. The eggs in the nest are my spiritual truths and your faith, which no one shall be allowed to steal from you. I watch over my own."** *No evil shall befall you, no affliction come near your tent. For God commands the angels to guard you in all your ways. With their hands they shall support you, lest you strike your foot against a stone. (Psalm 91:10-12)*

July 3
I called Miguel today and he sounds so much more energetic and hopeful! He is still doing many holistic things, finishing chemotherapy, and now taking some product that many people in his native Colombia are taking called Uzo™ by a company called Omnilife™. I've never heard of it, but he says they have had much success curing people of cancer by using the product over there. Wow! I am amazed at what God leads each person to. I am concerned though, because his doctor has advised him to stop some of the holistic procedures, claiming that they are dangerous for him because his white count is so low. We shall see. I judge nothing, but merely observe and pray. Time will tell.

I also called another lady, who had called me for help, to see how she is doing. She is going to the holistic clinic and also taking the Protocel™ formula. I am definitely going to follow these two and keep up with their progress. They have both prayed and asked for guidance. Bless them both, O Father.

And being on a roll, I called a third person. I am trying to help her friend who is considered terminal with cancer of the liver. But, her friend has become very attached to her comfort foods of french fries, sodas, etc., and very tied to traditional treatment. Only you, God, can work on that. I pray for your grace to be upon her. Amen.

July 4

Today is Independence Day. Thank you, Lord, for the freedom we have, that no other country has invaded us or has control over us. May you continue to be the God of our nation.

Lord, I wish to ask you a question that has been on my mind. My ultimate desire is to be one of your holy saints. How will I know that I am arriving at this? I want to stay healed and to go beyond healing.

"You have already learned the power of communication with me. Always remain in communication with me. You also are becoming more aware of the power of words, spoken, unspoken, and written. You know that good emanates forth from them, but they also have the potential for harm. The same is true of thoughts; they are unspoken words and images. One small sentence has great thunderous expression in the kingdom—words you say to yourself and your words or thoughts to and about others. Once words and thoughts are guarded and guided by me, everything changes—the glow of the spirit expands."

Two sentences came to me immediately as you spoke, Lord. The first had tremendous dire consequences for the entire world. It was, *The man I shall kiss is the one; arrest him and lead him away securely."(Mark 14:44)* This is the sentence that Judas spoke to inform the Sanhedrin that he would betray you, his friend, Jesus. The other sentence involves what you said on the cross with such mercy and tenderness, when you stated, *Father, forgive them, for they know not what they do. (Luke 23:31)* This helps me understand how powerful our words are, but I know I have not gotten complete self control in this area just yet. We Italians are used to blurting out verbally what we are thinking, immediately. Sometimes that is wonderful and spontaneous and sometimes it's a mood killer. Set a keeper at the gate of my mind, that it may not think the words to form sentences that might hurt you or others. Set another guard at the gate of my mouth so that my tongue will not utter what is not from you. *If anyone considers himself religious and yet does not keep a tight rein on his tongue, he deceives himself and his religion is worthless. (James 1:26)* Amen.

Heavenly Pearls of Wisdom

What you need is already prepared. It appears when you need it.

Recognize prayers answered. Sometimes you provide the answer to someone else or they provide it to you, through the Lord.

Look for the stories within the story. Both in scripture and in your daily life.

Sing God to you. He will sing back and draw you close.

Learn to recognize unholy suggestions. Once they are recognized, pray to send them away. Let no illusions become reality.

Guard words to yourself and others. Words are a powerful means of expression.

19
The Circle Completed

July 9
Lord, I am feeling an excitement about life now—an excitement about life that I've never felt before, like something really good is about to happen, in addition to the wonderment of being healed. I thank you for the feeling of joyful expectancy! I am looking at each person I see differently. I am blessing many others. I not only feel healed, but actually "squeaky clean." I cannot thank you enough. My heart sings. I am ready to leave the nest. You have prepared me. I trust you to keep the car running and help me with any necessary maintenance. Amen.

Keep the Car Running Smoothly

God has given me a new car (body). Do I need to continue with the heavy regimen to guarantee that the car doesn't rust, get decayed, or have a foul running engine? I will ask God for His guidance on this. Does this mean that I can eat, drink, and be overly merry with reckless abandon? I know God's answer will be "no". I can't treat my body like a car and peel out when accelerating, slam on the brakes when stopping, take curves at break-neck speeds, never put oil in the car, have fast food remnants on the floorboards, put in the cheapest gas, race with other drivers, and drive through fields and sand dunes as if I have a 4-wheel drive vehicle. Then, one day, the car just quits and I wonder what happened. (My biggest problem when I was young was running over curbs because I often misjudged the distance, or in a parking lot, forgot they were there!) So, it makes sense that I do need to keep the car in good shape, which is my body, to prevent "body abuse."

I will admit that I didn't always take the best care of my body. For a few years, when under great stress, I consumed at least 2 to 3 bottles of beer every evening to calm and "soothe" myself. *I was an untamed calf. If you allow me, I will return, for you are the Lord, my God. (Jeremiah 31:18)* Will I ever return to those kinds of harmful habits? No. Not if I expect my body to remain in good shape to fulfill the Lord's purpose.

The rule of thumb is 90/10. Eat well and drink nourishing liquids 90 percent of the time and "cheat" the other 10 percent. That means cheat a little bit, not a going crazy type of cheating. Our office had a Thanksgiving party and I ate everything, including one of each of the desserts. Ugh! I was so sick for the next two days. Now that is not cheating just a little bit. No more driving the car over curbs and expecting everything to stay in alignment.

It is now a habit for me to eat well, drink lots of distilled water, and green tea. It is easy to take calcium, magnesium, and potassium supplements every day. It is natural to eat fish, chicken, and turkey. It's fun going to Yoga and I can now keep up with the young ones and put a few of them in awe in that class. It takes a minimum of 21 days to establish a habit. I've been doing these things for over 2 years. It's beyond a habit. It's a lifestyle. And this lifestyle, along with staying connected with God, leads to an inner belief that all is well and will continue to be well.

July 11
Since I feed so many birds in the back yard, there are always loose feathers everywhere. Every day, I collect the feathers

that the birds have "donated" to me and put them in the back corner. I call it my feather garden. Of course, I see several of them disappear when I notice them being held in the beaks of another bird building a nest, but it's been a fun past time.

Today, I picked up a feather and hurriedly walked back to deposit it in the feather garden and the most fascinating thing happened. Instead of spiraling down to the ground, some sort of wind whisked it out of my hand, almost as if someone were taking it from me. The wind picked it up and carried it upward into the tree above my head and out of sight! That was pretty neat and had never happened before! I take that as an inspirational sign. I'm not getting weird. I enjoy life and what it brings. The feather flew up with no bird attached to it!

"To those who focus on me, many wonders occur. It is I showing you that anything is possible for your Lord. If someone approached you and said, 'It is possible for this feather to fly upwards attached to no bird', you would have denied it. Now you know with the simplest of acts, that wondrous things are possible in such ways that man cannot imagine. And so it is with all situations. When called upon with faith, each one will experience my love in wondrous and yet simple ways. And they will know—they will know it is I who perform these acts of love for them.

For you, it is also symbolic. I am lifting you lightly as a feather to new heights. At these heights, more is visible to your consciousness. Your spirit is healed. *Blessed are the poor in spirit, for theirs is the kingdom of Heaven. (Matthew 5:3)* **Yet, more blessed is the spirit who has found Me within. No longer are they poor in spirit but rich and full in spirit. You are now rich in spirit. Go forth and share that richness with others who seek it. Amen."**

Lord, thank you for your gentle guidance and beautiful ways. I feel so blessed to see you in the simple things. I will always be in awe of your power and yet your tenderness. Amen. *Happy those whom you guide, Lord, whom you teach by your instruction. (Psalm 94:12)*

July 11 (later in the day)

"You are coming to know me as the Lord of the New Testament, the new Covenant—a loving, humble, giving, and benevolent Being. The omnipresence includes being within you, acting out from you, as you. You have learned that I do not change with the wind, which blows in different directions. I am the God of constant Whispers and Roses. You have learned to lean on me and not on your own understanding. And most importantly, you know that I am the way, I am the solution, I am who I am. Amen."

I thank you for never changing, Lord. I thank you for your humble, gentle, giving nature. We overlook that beautiful part of you.

God Bows Before Us

As I heard God speak, the image came into my mind of God's humbleness. I saw a beautiful magnificent horse bow before a man. It bowed ever so slowly, gently, and gracefully, that my eyes filled with tears. This is how God humbles himself before us, his own creation! What kind of God loves his own people so much that he bows humbly before them? One who exhibits nothing but pure love. Pure love is impossible for us to fathom. Yet, it is available to us 24 hours of every day.

For God so loved the world that he gave his one and only Son, that whoever believes in him shall not perish, but have eternal life. (John 3:16) What kind of God comes to earth as a man and humbles himself to be an ordinary citizen, allows himself to be rebuked, called evil, chased out of the city, betrayed by a so-called friend, beaten, spit upon, and killed? I think I would have reached my limit of humbleness after the first rebuking from church elders. That's the kind of God I want to draw close to. That's the God that wants us to be well, happy, holy, powerful in His name, and in harmony.

In Max Lucado's book, *3:16 The Numbers of Hope,* he speaks extensively of the magnitude of the unearthly love of God for us, *agape* love. He states that we cannot win God's love, nor can we lose it. But, we can resist it, become blind, and refuse to accept it. He says that if God wants to touch you, let him![1]

God gave everyone a free will and they are allowed to choose to follow Him and His ways or not to follow Him. If they purposely choose not to follow Him, then they are choosing the opposite of everything He is. They are choosing the opposite of goodness, the opposite of mercy, the opposite of wellness. This becomes manifested as war, poverty, crime, and disease. *I said, O Lord, have mercy on me, heal me; for I have sinned against you. (Psalm 41:4)*

There are those who don't even realize that they have a choice and that by not deliberately choosing, they have allowed someone else or some other entity to choose for them. I was one of those for a long time. I never thought about making any kind of choice. I rocked along with the rest of the crowd. We are then unknowingly partakers of the thoughts and beliefs of others, either those who have good thoughts and choices or those who have bad thoughts and actions.

God humbles Himself before ALL—those who consciously choose and those who don't. I know that what saved me was making the choice to embrace this love and humbleness of the Lord. I felt it, I felt loved no matter what I had done in the past or who I thought I was. I felt God's humbleness when he offered me the rose of health. I, in turn, wanted to humble myself before His greatness and majesty. That connection with the Divine is what healed me and that connection is available to all, not just me. I thought it was everything I "did" to help myself, but God still had to be the one in charge. Period.

Go Forth in Confidence

July 12

"And now I say to you, recognize and revel in your oneness with Me. It is time to go forth with an unshakable peace

and confidence. When you have unshakable faith and confidence, nothing anyone says or does can torment you. *...we who are receiving the unshakable kingdom should have gratitude...(Hebrews 12:28)* **You will be confident that I work all things for your good. You will be confident in your decisions and direction. You will be confident that no disease or darkness can come up against you. You will be confident that I live out from you—confident of My never-ending love and presence. It is time. Amen"**

O, Lord. With your help I am arriving at that point of my life and my relationship with you. I ask this of you because only you can provide that confidence, just like you did to all of your disciples through the working of the Holy Spirit. I'm a little bit afraid to leave the nest, but you have said that it is time. I go forth. I trust you and your word. Amen. *Such confidence as this is ours through Christ before God. (2 Corinthians 3:4)*

It's time to go back out into the world with confidence. I do have confidence, but I'm going to continue to call upon God to make it full-time confidence. At first, it was what I call "on and off confidence", like a light switch with a dimmer control. It was on when I felt great, but it would try to go off when I felt any pain. It was on when everyone complimented my holistic approach and then someone would try to hit the dimmer switch of my confidence by attempting to negate the results. The confident switch was on when I sped through easy days and then flipped off if I had a rough day in any way. It is difficult to leave the confidence switch in the on position at all times, but the Lord assures us that He is there, granting us more confidence as we ask for it and are ready to receive it. *So, we are always courageous, although we know that while we are at home in the body we are away from the Lord, for we walk by faith and not by sight. (2 Corinthians 5:6-7)*

When people first asked me if I was healed, I hesitantly said yes. It was also usually followed by a "but I'm still feeling this" or "but I still worry about that." No more. Now I answer with a resounding and confident, "Yes, I am healed." I'm arriving at the place where nothing they respond with phases me one way or the other, because I know who is behind me 100 percent and within me. *We are his house, if only we hold fast to our confidence and pride in our hope. (Hebrews 3: 6)*

Even though I don't know where I'm heading, I'm going there with confidence because I know who is with me, leading and preparing the way. He is the same One who has prepared the way for you. When I make a decision, I have prayed about it, asked God to set the table before me, and now have the confidence that the decision is in accordance with His will. *The fruit of righteousness will be peace; the effect of righteousness will be quietness and confidence forever. (Isaiah 32:17)*

July 13
Lord, this book is finished. I feel that it's time to bring the story to a happy end—that you have no more to say for this endeavor. I look to you for guidance. Walk with me, Lord.
"My words to you are only the start. I have need of you in other places and endeavors. You have been reborn. You are a new creation. And in being reborn, the circle is completed. Amen ." *...but because of his mercy, he saved us through the bath of rebirth and renewal by the Holy Spirit. (Titus 3:5)*

July 14
Even though it's 102 degrees today, I'm sitting outside with a slight breeze blowing and just enjoying being able to rest awhile. Snickers, my miracle cat, is at my feet and I've been petting him as he purrs. He sure doesn't sweat like I do. Oh, I mean he doesn't detoxify quite as well as I'm doing. I'm sipping my distilled water and pretending it's tea with mint. My wilting basil plant is next to me on the patio. Maybe I'll put a sprig of it in my water and see how that tastes. Life is good.

I am free. I hear the neighbor's donkey braying and I know all is indeed well and in Divine right order. Ah, Thank you God.

Let what you heard from the beginning remain in you. If what you heard from the beginning remains in you, then you will remain in the Son and in the Father. And this is the promise that he made us: eternal life. (1 John 2:24-25)

Heavenly Pearls of Wisdom

Keep the car running. By remaining in contact with the Lord and being moderate in all manner of eating and drinking.

Revere God's Humbleness. When you realize what He continues to do out of humbleness for you, your heart will ache for Him.

Grab the Confidence and go. Ask for confidence in healing and staying healed. Take that confidence and proceed forward!

Enjoy every simple thing. Just enjoy it, see God all around you, and feel His presence within you, the beautiful rose.

"When you need me,
I am here,
Through joy and sorrow,
Today and tomorrow.
Never ending."

References

Chapter 2 – Into the Darkness

1. Russell, A.J. (editor), *God Calling,* (1978), Berkley Publishing Group, New York, ISBN 0-515-09026-3, pages 137-138

2. Anderson, Greg, *Cancer: 50 Essential Things to Do,* (1999), Penguin Putnam Inc., New York, ISBN 0-452-28074-5, pages 8, 44-45

3. Ibid, page 174

Chapter 3 – A Shaft of Light

1. O'Donnell, Michele Longo, *Of Monkeys and Dragons: Freedom from the Tyranny of Disease,* (2002 Second Printing), La Vida Press, Boerne

2. St. Teresa of Avila, *The Interior Castle,* translation by Mirabai Starr, (2003), Riverhead Books, New York, ISBN 1-57322-248-8, page 35

3. Dr. Lorraine Day-*www.drday.com*

4. Trigiani, Adriana, *Milk Glass Moon,* (2002), Ballantine Books, New York, ISBN-0-345-44585-6, page 204.

5. Myss, Caroline, *Entering the Castle: An Inner Path to God and Your Soul*, (2007), Simon and Schuster, New York, ISBN -13: 978-0-7432-5532-5

Chapter 4 – Appearance of Grace

1. Goldsmith, Joel. *The Master Speaks,* (2004 Second Printing), Acropolis Books, Lakewood, Colorado. ISBN 1-889051-42-X, page 97

2. Weil, Andrew. *Breathing: The Master Key to Self Healing*, (2000) ISBN-13: 978-1564557261

Chapter 5 – Finding the Lord

1. *A Christmas Story,* Director Bob Clark, Peter Bilingsley, Darrin McGavin, Release 18 November 1983, USA, Christmas Tree Films

2. O'Donnell, Michele Longo, *The God That We've Created,* (2005) La Vida Press, Boerne, ISBN 0-9676861-4-8

3. Yance, Donald, *Herbal Medicine, Healing, and Cancer: A Comprehensive Program for Prevention and Treatment,* (1999) McGraw-Hill New York, ISBN 0-87983-968-6, pages 53-56, 88

Chapter 6 – Fullness of Grace

1. *Willy Wonka and the Chocolate Factory,* Director Mel Stuart, Gene Wilder, Jack Albertson, Peter Ostrum, Release 30 June 1971, USA, David L. Wolper Produtions

Chapter 7 – God's Grace Flows

1. St. Teresa of Avila, *The Interior Castle,* translation by Mirabai Starr, (2003), Riverhead Books, New York, (2004) ISBN 1-57322-248-8, pages 15, 30

2. Unknown, *The Cloud of Unknowing,* Tom Griffith, Editor, (2005), Wordsworth Editions Limited, ISBN 1-84022-126-7, pages 103-104

3. Byrne, Rhonda, *The Secret,* (2006), Beyond Words Publishing, Hillsboro, ISBN 13: 978-1-58270-170-7, pages 141-153

4. Hay, Louise, *You Can Heal Your Life,* (1999), Hay House, Inc., ISBN 13: 978-1-56170-628-0, page 63

5. Quillin, Patrick, PhD, with Noreen Quillin, *Beating Cancer With Nutrition,* (2005 Revised Edition), Nutrition Times Press, Inc., Carlsbad, California ISBN 978-0-9638372-9-5, pages 9, 13, 15.

Chapter 8 – The Manifestation of God

1. Quillin, Patrick, PhD, with Noreen Quillin, *Beating Cancer With Nutrition,* (2005 Revised Edition), Nutrition Times Press, Inc., Carlsbad, California ISBN 978-0-9638372-9-5, pages 117-119

2. O'Donnell, Michele Longo, *Of Monkeys and Dragons: Freedom from the Tyranny of Disease,* (2002 Second Printing), La Vida Press, Boerne, ISBN 0-9676861-1-3, pages 211-220

3. Ibid

4. Berendt, John, *The City of Falling Angels,* (2005), Penguin, New York, ISBN 0-14303-693-9, page 116, 117-123

5. Ibid, page 388

Chapter 9 – Channel of Grace

1. Merton, Thomas, *The Seven Storey Mountain; An Autobiography of Faith,* (1976), Harcourt, Austin, ISBN 13: 978-0-15-601086-3, page 254

2. Ibid

3. Quillin, Patrick, PhD, with Noreen Quillin, *Beating Cancer With Nutrition,* (2005 Revised Edition), Nutrition Times Press, Inc., Carlsbad, California ISBN 978-0-9638372-9-5, page339-342

4. Information on Dr. Gonzalez- *www.the-moneychanger.com:80/articles_files/health/dr_nicholas_gonzalez.phtml*

5. Pierce, Tanya Harter, *Outsmart Your Cancer: Alternative Non-Toxic Treatments That Work,(2007) 4th printing,* Thoughtworks Publishing, Stateline, Nevada. ISBN-13: 978-0-9728867-3-4, pages 200-207

6. Information on Dr. Gonzalez- *www.the-moneychanger.com:80/articles_files/health/dr_nicholas_gonzalez.phtml*

7. Faloon, William, "Ending the Atrocities", *Life Extension,* (2009), Volume 15, (3), March, LE Publications, Inc., pages 7-12.

8. Pierce, Tanya Harter, *Outsmart Your Cancer: Alternative Non-Toxic Treatments That Work,(2007) 4th printing,* Thoughtworks Publishing, Stateline, Nevada. ISBN-13: 978-0-9728867-3-4. pages 65-70, 73-79

Chapter 10 – Mercy of the Lord

1. Goldsmith, Joel. *The Master Speaks,* (2004 Second Printing), Acropolis Books, Lakewood, Colorado. ISBN 1-889051-42-X, page 145

2. Balch, Dr. James and Balch, Phyllis. *Prescription for Nutritional Healing,* 3rd edition (2000), Avery, ISBN-13: 978-1583330777, page 545-547

3. Information on Dr. Gonzalez- *www.the-moneychanger.com:80/articles_files/health/dr_nicholas_gonzalez.phtml*

4. Kloss, Jethro, *Back to Eden,* (2005), Lotus Press, Twin Lakes, ISBN-10: 978-0-9409-8510-0, pages 862-865

5. *http://www.lawbuzz.com/famous_trials/erin_brockovich/erin_brockovich.htm*

6. Merton, Thomas, *The Seven Storey Mountain; An Autobiography of Faith,* (1976), Harcourt, Austin, ISBN 13: 978-0-15-601086-3

7. Ibid

8. Goldsmith, Joel. *The Master Speaks,* (2004 Second Printing) , Acropolis Books, Lakewood, Colorado. ISBN 1-889051-42-X, page 36

Chapter 11 – Beyond the Earthly Senses

1. Hay, Louise, *You Can Heal Your Life,* Hay House, Inc., (1999), ISBN 13: 978-1-56170-628-0, pages 174, 214

Chapter 12 – God's Mission Revealed

1. Mother Teresa: *No Greater Love,* (2000), MJF Books ISBN-13: 978-1567314014, page 88

2. Merton, Thomas, *The Seven Storey Mountain; An Autobiography of Faith,* Harcourt, Austin, (1976). ISBN 13: 978-0-15-601086-3, page 260-261

3. Mother Teresa: *No Greater Love,* (2000), MJF Books ISBN-13: 978-1567314014, page 54

4. Pierce, Tanya Harter, *Outsmart Your Cancer: Alternative Non-Toxic Treatments That Work,(2007) 4th printing,* Thoughtworks Publishing, Stateline, Nevada. ISBN-13: 978-0-9728867-3-4, page 96

5. *http://www.craniosacraltherapy.org*

Chapter 14 – Renewal of Spirit

1. Pope John Paul II, *Crossing the Threshold of Hope,* (1994), Alfred Knopf Inc., New York, ISBN 0-679-44058-5, Page 17

2. Cavallini, Guliana, *Things Visible and Invisible: Images of the Spirituality of St. Catherine of Siena,* (2001), Alba House, New York, ISBN 0-8189-0733-9, Pages 9-16

Chapter 15 – The Flower Blooms

1. Merton, Thomas, *The Seven Storey Mountain; An Autobiography of Faith,* (1976), Harcourt, Austin. ISBN 13: 978-0-15-601086-3, page 424

Chapter 16 – Changed Forever

1. Young, Robert O., PhD, and Shelley Redford Young, *The pH Miracle; Balance Your Diet, Reclaim Your Health,* (2002) Wellness Central, New York, ISBN 10: 446-53619-9, page 7

2. Pierce, Tanya Harter, *Outsmart Your Cancer: Alternative Non-Toxic Treatments That Work,(2007) 4th printing,* Thoughtworks Publishing, Stateline, Nevada. ISBN-13: 978-0-9728867-3-4, page 269

3. Young, Robert O., PhD, and Shelley Redford Young, *The pH Miracle; Balance Your Diet, Reclaim Your Health,* (2002) Wellness Central, New York, ISBN 10: 446-53619-9, page 19, 37-38, 22

4. Quillin, Patrick, PhD, with Noreen Quillin, *Beating Cancer With Nutrition,* (2005 Revised Edition), Nutrition Times Press, Inc., Carlsbad, California ISBN 978-0-9638372-9-5, page 39-40

Chapter 17 – Light Unto the Darkness

1. Pierce, Tanya Harter, *Outsmart Your Cancer: Alternative Non-Toxic Treatments That Work, (2007) 4th printing,* Thoughtworks Publishing, Stateline, Nevada. ISBN-13: 978-0-9728867-3-4, pages 125-198

Chapter 18 – Arriving at a New Place

1. *Australia,* Director Baz Luhrmann,Nicole Kidman, Hugh Jackman, Release 26 November 2008, USA, Bazmark Films.

2. *Madagascar 2: Escape to Africa*, Directors Erin Darnell and Tom McGrath, Ben Stiller, Chris Rock, David Schwimmer, Relaease 7 November 2008, USA, DreamWorks Animation.

Chapter 19 – The Circle Completed

1. Lucado, Max, *3:16: The Numbers of Hope,* (2007), Thomas Nelson, Inc., Nashville, ISBN 10: 0-8499-0193-6, page 39

Bibliography and Recommended Reading List

Anderson, Greg, *Cancer: 50 Essential Things to Do,* Penguin Putnam Inc., New York, (1999), ISBN 0-452-28074-5

Benenate, Becky and Durepos, Joseph, Editors, *No Greater Love: Mother Teresa,* Barnes and Noble Books, New York. (1997) ISBN 1-56731-401-5

Berendt, John, *The City of Falling Angels,* Penguin, New York, (2005), ISBN 0-14303-693-9

*Byrne, Rhonda, *The Secret,* Beyond Words Publishing, Hillsboro, (2006), ISBN 13: 978-1-58270-170-7

Cavallini, Guliana, *Things Visible and Invisible: Images of the Spirituality of St. Catherine of Siena,* Alba House, New York, (2001), ISBN 0-8189-0733-9

Faloon, William, "Ending the Atrocities", *Life Extension,* Volume 15, (3), March, LE Publications, Inc., (2009).

Goldsmith, Joel. *The Master Speaks,* Acropolis Books, Lakewood, Colorado. (2004 Second Printing) ISBN 1-889051-42-X

Haanel, Charles, *The Master Key System,* Wilder Publications, LLC, Radford, (2007), ISBN 10: 1-934451-32-0

*Hay, Louise, *You Can Heal Your Life,* Hay House, Inc., (1999), ISBN 13: 978-1-56170-628-0

Kloss, Jethro, *Back to Eden,* Lotus Press, Twin Lakes, (2005), ISBN-10: 978-0-9409-8510-0

Lucado, Max, *3:16: The Numbers of Hope,* Thomas Nelson, Inc., Nashville, (2007), ISBN 10: 0-8499-0193-6

Merton, Thomas, *The Seven Storey Mountain; An Autobiography of Faith,* Harcourt, Austin, (1976). ISBN 13: 978-0-15-601086-3

*Myss, Caroline, *Entering the Castle: An Inner Path to God and Your Soul*, Simon and Schuster, New York, (2007), ISBN -13: 978-0-7432-5532-5

Odell, Catherine, *Faustina: Apostle of Divine Mercy,* Our Sunday Visitor Publishing Division, Huntington, (1998), ISBN 0-87973-923-1

*O'Donnell, Michele Longo, *Of Monkeys and Dragons: Freedom from the Tyranny of Disease,* La Vida Press, Boerne, (2002 Second Printing), ISBN 0-9676861-1-3

*O'Donnell, Michele Longo, *The God That We've Created, the Basic Cause of All Disease,* La Vida Press, Boerne, (2005) ISBN0-9676861-4-8

*O'Donnell, Michele Longo, *When the Wolf is at the Door: The Simplicity of Healing,* La Vida Press, Boerne, (2007), ISBN 978-0-9814649-0-9

*Pierce, Tanya Harter, *Outsmart Your Cancer: Alternative Non-Toxic Treatments That Work, (2007) 4th printing,* Thoughtworks Publishing, Stateline, Nevada. ISBN-13: 978-0-9728867-3-4

Pope John Paul II, *Crossing the Threshold of Hope,* (1994), Alfred Knopf Inc., New York, ISBN 0-679-44058-5

*Quillin, Patrick, PhD, with Noreen Quillin, *Beating Cancer With Nutrition,* Nutrition Times Press, Inc., Carlsbad, California (2005 Revised Edition), ISBN 978-0-9638372-9-5

*Russell, A.J. (editor), *God Calling,* Berkley Publishing Group, New York, (1978), ISBN 0-515-09026-3

Savard, Liberty, *Shattering Your Strongholds,* Bridge-Logos Publishers, North Brunswick, (1997 Fifth Printing), ISBN 0-88270-713-2

St. Teresa of Avila, *The Interior Castle,* translation by Mirabai Starr, (2003),, Riverhead Books, New York, (2004) ISBN 1-57322-248-8

The New American Bible, World Bible Publishers, Inc., Iowa Falls, (1991)

Thomas, Richard, *The Essiac Report: Canada's Remarkable Unknown Cancer Remedy,* (1993) Alternative Treatment Network, Los Angeles, ISBN 0-9639818-0-3

Unknown, *The Cloud of Unknowing,* Tom Griffith, Editor, Wordsworth Editions Limited, (2005), ISBN 1-84022-126-7

Yance, Donald, *Herbal Medicine, Healing, and Cancer: A Comprehensive Program for Prevention and Treatment,* (1999) McGraw-Hill, New York, ISBN 0-87983-968-6

*Young, Robert O., PhD, and Shelley Redford Young, *The pH Miracle; Balance Your Diet, Reclaim Your Health,* (2002) Wellness Central, New York, ISBN 10: 446-53619-9

**These are highly recommended to begin the journey toward health.*

Web Sites and Other Information

http://www.Biblegateway.com (scripture quotes)

Diet of rats-*http://science.jrank.org/pages/5748/Rats-Diet.html*

Information on Dr. Gonzalez- *http://www.themoneychanger.com:80/articles_files/health/dr_nicholas_gonzalez.phtml*

Dr. Lorraine Day-*http://www.drday.com*

Life Extension Foundation— *http://www.lef.org*

Cranio Sacral Therapy— *http://www.craniosacraltherapy.org*

Order Sons of Italy-*http://www.osia.org*

Japanese Green Tea—*http://www.hggreentea@yahoo.com* (Haraki-Gordon Green Tea Imports)

Living Beyond Disease (associated with the Boerne Clinic, below) *http://www.livingbeyonddisease.com* 1-830-755-8767

Holistic Health Care Center, 107 Scenic Loop Road, Boerne, Texas 78006, 1-830-755-6420

Acknowledgments

My first acknowledgement is to my Lord and Savior.

Abundant thanks to my family: my wonderful and supportive husband Lloyd, daughters Angela and Andraya, son-in-laws Dustin and Derek, my father and mother, Louis and Donna Fidone, all my brothers and sisters, Jerry, David, James, Joann and their families. Their contributions are too numerous to count. The Griggs family of folks, Elizabeth Griggs Whitehead and husband Frank, Scott and Susan Griggs, David and Cheryl Griggs, all of the Marx family. Chad, Lori, Madison, and Rylee Pierce, Jan Payne Pierce, and Gaylene Boman (Moms of Derek and Dustin).

Extreme gratefulness is given to the Holistic Health Care Clinic: Michele Longo O'Donnell who inspired me to healing and greater holiness, Melissa Raymond who encouraged me, her husband Phil Raymond who initiated this book, and Caitlin Raymond who is just all around fun, Rosie Arredondo who laughs a lot, Priscilla Geister who gave me my first treatment, along with Brenda Hernandez, Carmen Hernandez, Gracie Santos, Vicky Ramos, Ana Padron, who all provided treatment and comfort, and fellow patients and families.

To the Sons of Italy Organization, Pompeo Coppini Lodge members Gaitano (Tom) Butera who introduced me to the holistic clinic, Diana Grippi who came to the hospital and my home for metaphysical healing, Sam Bernadino who made me laugh hysterically in the hospital, Jean Paletta, Marguerite Casella, Tinker Butera Kochwelp, Dr. Anthony and Susan Sabino for helping me find my "voice" in writing , Dr. David and Toni O'Mara, Dr. Edward Scavone, Joanna Hansen, Lance Gunderson, Margie and Eddie Wood, Dr. Clementina Geiser, Raymond Botello, Dr. Joe and Frances Bevilacqua, Jerry and Pat DuTerroil, George W. and Dr. Alice De Rosa, Steve and Suzi Rizzo, Dave and Rose Anderson, Betty Berchelmann,

Camille Fiorillo, Luciana Cristadoro who is my Italian teacher and her husband Francesco, and all those who gave me encouragement and inspiration.

For your tough spirit to Larry and Kim Johnson, Bob and Linda Bason. Many thanks to our favorite restauranteur, Vic Pisano of Macaroni Grill, for his generosity and support.

A big hug to my boss, Rick Brown, who visited me in the hospital even though he hates them, and friends at Realty Executives, his wife Mavis Brown, Kyle Brown, Ricky Brown, Karen Critchlow, Sam Schifano, Jessica Lantz, Lucy Biltoft, Manuel Acero, Manny Arredondo, Smitty Salinas, Kathy Smith, Nora Roberts, Dana LeSueur, Nora Carmona, Jim Dawson, Gracie Santos, Robert Sanchez, and Jordan Williams.

My friends from Northside Independent School District, Margaret and Don Christilles, Becky and John Nick, Linda Hanson, Marilyn Redding, Jan Henderson, Nancy Harper-Smith and Judy Joseph who juiced the first vegetables ever for me, Jeanne Schattenberg, Pearl Hedlund, Judy Harris, Brenda Rasberry, Linda Hansen-Masters, Harriette Spires, Mary Moulder, Dr. Carlota Dwyer, Carol Mayo, Pam Brenner, Pat Albrecht, Frances Gonzales, Betty Puckett, Ruth Leal, Priscilla Lurz and all of the Grady's prayer group, Shirley Ferguson, Bonnie Ellison, and Norma Rabago of NISD Partnerships, Cipriano and Cathy Munoz, Barbara Friedson, Pat and Jim Davis, Kay Ingram, Donna and Jim Martin, Bruce and Janis Tschoepe, Ruth Wolf, Melinda Diaz, Dennis Alexander, Judy Christians, Sheryl Parker, Donna Miller, Judy Enderlin, Pat Burrier, Marie Maddox, Kay Manna, Sharon Solanik, Suzy Groff, Gail Ellison, Carolyn Lecocke, Kathy Phillips, Peggy Tindall, Peggy Escue, Lorraine Trawick, and Mary Cavanaugh who all helped me in so many ways.

Abundant blessings on all of my cousins who provided support, Lucia Catania, Beverly Hazuka, Debbie Synowicki, Mary and John Fidone, James and Galyn Lacewell, Jody and Link Lacewell,

Cyndie and Dr. Bruce Hartzell, Carmelo, Assunta, Gabriele, and Giacomo Fidone of Sicily.

Thanks to Daryl and Diane Dilworth, Harriette Palmer, Barbara and Jimmy Green, my Godmother and aunt Phyllis De-Carlo, who sent tons of letters of support and prayers, Lynn and Katie Jackson, Pat and Walter Nielsen, Ruth Hernandez, Michael Idrogo, Eric and Christy Cracraft, David Barerro, Wayne Sihrer, Vicky Zapf who introduced me to Essiac Tea, Ernie Truitt, Pauline Chapman, Lonnie Shuler, Nita Mastin of Frost Bank, Dave and Clara Schorg, Pat Wood, Carol Kraft, Dora Copeland, Jane Adams who knitted me a cap for my cold head and a prayer shawl, Nicole Townsley, fellow retreatant Pamela Hood, Jessica Land, my pal from the Science Center Jackie Gandre, our attorney Johnny Lane for his encouraging words, Dora Postiglione and family from Barletta, Italy, my master's degree classmate, Dr. Joanna Ponce-Gonzalez and hubby Speedy, Virgie Mireles, my hairdresser Susie Perez who tried to make me look like I had more hair during chemo, Danielle Brown who shared her book experience and poetry, Mike, Pam, Paris, and Pia Taylor, Kathy Gruber, Reverend Steve Cottingham who prayed with us before surgery in the hospital, Roy and Ellie Latigo, John Garza who prayed over me.

My friends from church, Jori and Mary Nell Zabava, Jay and Lisa Gabrelcik, George and Cindy Munoz, Rita Logan, Teresa, Katie, and Jessica Hottenstein, Gennell Slay, Charles McCarthy, Susie Montgomery, Dave and Patti Tuttle, Paul and Margaret Cwiklik, who sent cards and provided prayers and support every week.

My appreciation to my clients present and past, Luis and Lisa Bocanegra, Jane, Toni, and Steve Watkins, Olwen Pierce-Smith, Jim and Heidi Webb, Ike and Cindy Wilkerson, Kevin Pellone and Dawn Oerichbauer, Tom and Tomala Gueringer, Matthew, Les, Donna, and Emily Kuglics, Bill and Donna Carder, and Kevin, Tammy, Jessica, and Sharon Mauldin for their patience, understanding, and prayers. Gratitude for offerings of food and transportation goes to

First American Title Insurance Company with Nancy and Christy Janysek, and Lisa Shortner.

I am also thankful for my neighbors Keith, Carrie, and K.C. Holderfield, Michelle Keller, David and Rose Marie Frohn, Bill and Ellie Lester,Red Hat Society Members Mary Parris, Karron Dunlap, Gay Cooper, Victoria Tout, and Janice Bruno.

To Cheryl Brown and the staff of Brian Buffini and Company, who sent me encouraging cards, is extended my gratitude for thoughts and prayers across the miles.

To Lloyd's fellow police officers who showed tremendous compassion and visited me in the hospital such as Eddie and Ilda Gonzales, George and Juanita Ward, Terri Neal who gave me her pin to wear, Charles Marcus who was willing to lend a hand, and Andy Rodriguez who adjusted Lloyd's work schedule to allow hospital time with me.

To the prayer group at Ira First Baptist Church whom I have never met, but who prayed for me, I am grateful and overwhelmed with goodness to them including Leona Wiggins, Jerry Stokes, Jay and Faye Gernandt, Joe and Rhonda Falk, Jane McCarty, Raye Sterling, Ruby Johnson, Lonice Hall, Jean Sterling, Clyde Brown, Vicki L., Keith and Carla Clements, Shane, DeDe, Ashton, and Jordan Smith, Kenneth and Barbara Martin, Carla Sanchez, Hubert Clements, Billy and Verline Calley, Darryl and Teena Calley.

My warm thanks to Region 20 Education Service center and all my friends there including Ed and Connie Vara, Jan Dunevant, Judy Castleberry, Pat Sanders, Steve Peterson, Michelle Mika DeAtley, Linda and Phil Mason, and Louise Scanlon.

The understanding and care of my fellows at the University of Texas at San Antonio including my boss, Dr. Betty Merchant who provided much intellectual and mental support when I needed it most, Dr. Bruce Barnett, Dr. Alan Shoho, Dr. Betty Murakami and husband Bruce Barker who read Bible passages to me in the hospital and brought me a tape player, Lisa Chavez, Dr. Raymond and Mary Padilla who prayed with me, Dr. David Thompson, Dr. Page Smith, and Dr. Maricela Oliva.

Special thanks to the Living Beyond Disease ministry: Phil Raymond for starting me down this road and helping tremendously, Lee Lanning and Angela Sparks for tireless hours in editing, and Michele O'Donnell for suggestions and corrections.

No amount of acknowledgement would ever compensate for all that the above named have done for me. Many people brought food, took me to treatments, prayed, sent cards, visited me at home or in the hospital, called on the phone, helped me with juicing, cleaned vegetables, put me on prayer lists, shared recipes, gave enormous help with this book, and so many other valuable ways in which they lifted my spirit. My apologies to anyone I forgot. I am eternally grateful.

About the Author

Diana feels that she is an ordinary person who has been given an extraordinary assignment by the Lord. Her mission is to share her personal story of healing from cancer, spread the truth as it has been revealed to her, and to give others hope and life.

Diana holds a doctoral degree in education and the sciences from Texas A&M University in College Station, Texas. Her extensive background includes teaching research methods and philosophy to graduate students at the University of Texas in San Antonio, as well as teaching Human Anatomy at the University of Texas Health Science Center. She expanded her teaching into the high school arena and became an instructor of Biology, Chemistry, and Health Care Sciences for Northside Independent School District (NISD).

She became an administrator and served as principal of the Health Careers Academy in Edgewood Independent School District (EISD), followed by Director of Careers and Technology at both Edgewood and later, Northside ISD, from which she is now retired. Up until the creation of this book, she has been working as a real estate agent with her husband Lloyd.

The medical field has been graced by her work as a medical technologist and laboratory scientist in both the hospital and research facility settings. This background gave her insight into the treatments that she received, as well as the physiology of how supplements and herbs work in the body.

Numerous seminars on a variety of topics have been conducted by Diana during her tenure with the Region 20 Education Service Center. She states that the spiritual insights came from reading the Bible and the teachings of others, but most importantly, from the Lord Himself. The current focus of her seminars, speaking engagements, and other endeavors is to tell her story, provide encouragement, useful information, and spiritual guidance to others seeking healing and wellness.

Give the Gift of

Whispers & Roses

A Journal of Healing from Cancer

To Your Family, Friends, and Colleagues

Order Form

To order copies of Whispers & Roses by phone, call 1-877-445-4179.

To order copies online, go to *www.WhispersandRoses.com*

To order by fax, copy this form and fax to 1-830-755-6421

To order by mail, copy this form and mail to:
La Vida Press, 107 Scenic Loop Rd. Boerne, Texas 78006

Please send me ________ copies for a total of: $__________________
Sales Tax: (Texas residents only) 8.25% $__________________
Shipping: $5.95 for 1st book; $1.50 per additional: total $__________________
(All books shipped USPS)

TOTAL: $__________________
(All prices in U.S. dollars)

My check or money order is enclosed. Payable to La Vida Press.

Please charge my: Visa Mastercard Discover American Express

Name ____

Address ____

City/State/Zip _______________________________________

Phone __________________ Email __________________________

Card # ____ Exp Date __________

Signature_______________________________________ Security Code ______

For larger or wholesale orders, please call La Vida Press at 1-877-445-4179.